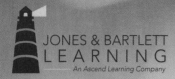

Information Systems for the Health Care Industry

Simulated Health Records Simplified

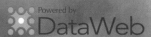

World Headquarters
Jones & Bartlett Learning
5 Wall Street
Burlington, MA 01803
978-443-5000
info@jblearning.com
www.jblearning.com

Jones & Bartlett Learning books and products are available through most bookstores and online booksellers. To contact Jones & Bartlett Learning directly, call 800-832-0034, fax 978-443-8000, or visit our website, www.jblearning.com.

Substantial discounts on bulk quantities of Jones & Bartlett Learning publications are available to corporations, professional associations, and other qualified organizations. For details and specific discount information, contact the special sales department at Jones & Bartlett Learning via the above contact information or send an email to specialsales@jblearning.com.

The content, statements, views, and opinions herein are the sole expression of the respective authors and not that of Jones & Bartlett Learning, LLC. Reference herein to any specific commercial product, process, or service by trade name, trademark, manufacturer, or otherwise does not constitute or imply its endorsement or recommendation by Jones & Bartlett Learning, LLC and such reference shall not be used for advertising or product endorsement purposes. All trademarks displayed are the trademarks of the parties noted herein. *Simulated Health Records Simplified* is an independent publication and has not been authorized, sponsored, or otherwise approved by the owners of the trademarks or service marks referenced in this product.

There may be images in this book that feature models; these models do not necessarily endorse, represent, or participate in the activities represented in the images. Any screenshots in this product are for educational and instructive purposes only. Any individuals and scenarios featured in the case studies throughout this product may be real or fictitious, but are used for instructional purposes only.

The authors, editor, and publisher have made every effort to provide accurate information. However, they are not responsible for errors, omissions, or for any outcomes related to the use of the contents of this book and take no responsibility for the use of the products and procedures described. Treatments and side effects described in this book may not be applicable to all people; likewise, some people may require a dose or experience a side effect that is not described herein. Drugs and medical devices are discussed that may have limited availability controlled by the Food and Drug Administration (FDA) for use only in a research study or clinical trial. Research, clinical practice, and government regulations often change the accepted standard in this field. When consideration is being given to use of any drug in the clinical setting, the health care provider or reader is responsible for determining FDA status of the drug, reading the package insert, and reviewing prescribing information for the most up-to-date recommendations on dose, precautions, and contraindications, and determining the appropriate usage for the product. This is especially important in the case of drugs that are new or seldom used.

This publication is designed to provide accurate and authoritative information in regard to the Subject Matter covered. It is sold with the understanding that the publisher is not engaged in rendering legal, accounting, or other professional service. If legal advice or other expert assistance is required, the service of a competent professional person should be sought.

Production Credits

Publisher: William Brottmiller
Executive Editor: Cathy L. Esperti
Technology Product Manager: Laurie K. Davis
Associate Editor: Teresa Reilly
Associate Director of Production: Julie Champagne Bolduc
Production Editors: Jill Morton and Joanna Lundeen
Marketing Manager: Grace Richards

VP, Manufacturing and Inventory Control: Therese Connell
Composition: Cenveo Publisher Services
Cover Design: Scott Moden
Cover Image: © Yellow/ShutterStock, Inc.
Printing and Binding: Courier Companies
Cover Printing: Courier Companies

To order this product, use ISBN: 978-1-284-03185-0

ISBN: 978-1-284-03186-7

6048

Printed in the United States of America

17 16 15 14 13   10 9 8 7 6 5 4 3 2 1

CONTENTS

INTRODUCTION

The VariPoint electronic health record learning portal is a Web-based software application designed for people who want to learn the basic functions and operation of a computer-based electronic health record system.

Course content has been developed to introduce users to the basic functions of an electronic health record software application with a particular focus on Patient Notes and Orders and Standards.

Electronic Health Records Defined

Electronic health record (EHR) systems are the electronic storage of patient medical information, including medical history, patient notes, and orders for procedures and treatments. They have several benefits. First, they provide decision support services for medical professionals and their patients. Second, they protect patients' privacy by segregating access to patient information based upon role and need to know. Third, they electronically interact with third-party service providers to exchange health and billing information. Finally, they provide healthcare providers and organizations the opportunity to determine and monitor health trends through data analytics. In summary, EHR systems offer an opportunity for increased efficiency, security, data analytics, and monitoring.

When This Workbook Is Most Useful

This workbook and access to the VariPoint Electronic Health Record application are most useful for users who want to familiarize themselves with the basic operation and function of an electronic health record software. We do not intend to limit our focus to students in a nursing program or allied health fields or health administration. Rather, any user who has an interest in learning about the core functionality of an electronic health record application and who wishes to develop an understanding of how the acceptance of this technology will transform how business is done in the healthcare industry can benefit from these materials. We purposefully have not loaded up this EHR with vendor-specific features, which we believe would distract from the user learning about the basic or core responsibilities of an EHR.

At its core, electronic health records can provide a range of benefits for healthcare providers, the payer community, and patients. First and foremost, electronic health records will allow healthcare providers access to information they need to deliver the best care possible. Doctors and other providers will have easy access to patient medical histories at any time during the course of their relationship. Furthermore, an electronic health record system will give providers ready access to all manner of decision support tools that will assist them in both diagnosing and treating patient medical problems. Two of these "decision support tools" are presented in this workbook. The system represented in this workbook places an emphasis on the important role of information security. The user will learn firsthand how patient medical records are brought together to the point-of-care and are still protected and managed in a clinical setting.

How This Workbook Is Organized

This workbook contains four Key Learning Assets organized into four chapters.

First and foremost, it contains instructions on how to access and use the online VariPoint Electronic Health Record application. This EHR is built using the powerful DataWeb Cloud Database Technology that is integrated into Microsoft's SQL Relational Database. You will be working with release 2.2. The EHR itself respects the data structure found in the VistA EHR, which has been in use at the Veterans Hospitals across the country for more than 15 years.

Second, you will find the Quick Start Guide and the annotated help screens, which are helpful in understanding the context in which EHRs operate.

Third, in addition to being able to create your own patient appointments and records, you will have full access to authentic patient medical histories. These records are fully de-personalized. This will give you a reasonably sized database of patient medical records in order to experience the search functions that are part of the operation of this EHR.

Finally, you will find a series of self-paced learning exercises that you can use to further extend your working understanding of EHRs. These learning exercises focus on Patient Notes and Orders and Medical Standards and reflect the Meaningful Use requirements of the HITECH Act of 2010.

We hope you find these resources helpful as you further your understanding of EHRs and the impact they will have on this fast-paced and extremely important industry.

SECTION 1

Getting Registered and Gaining Access

Registering as a User

This guide is designed to help users register for the system and begin using it immediately. It is accessible by clicking the registration link embedded in the email you received following the redemption of your course access code. Next, create a username and password that will be used to gain access to the Electronic Health Record (EHR) application, as shown below.

Register as a varipoint.com User

To get started, fill out the fields below. Enter your email address and a user name (without spaces) that you'll use to log on to varipoint.com.

Email:	jblDemoWed@Bizwebsolutions.net
User Name:	jblDemoWed
	e.g. John_Doe
Choose Password:	
Verify Password:	

☐ I have read and agree to the varipoint.com Member Agreement.* required

[Register]

Check the Member Agreement box to register. You will be taken to the My Account page, where the Simulated Health Records Simplified Course is displayed, along with any other Jones & Bartlett courses you might have. Click the course name, and the course logon page is presented for your username and password; click Secure Signin to enter the EHR.

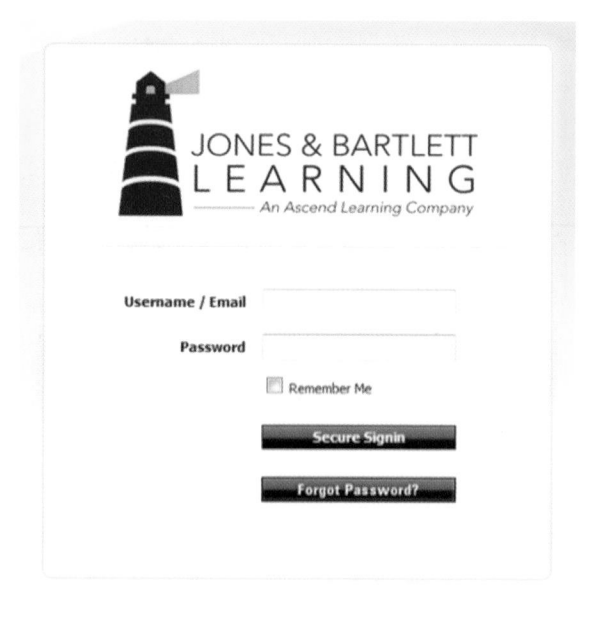

Need More Help?

Once you are in the EHR system, every screen has screen-sensitive help, accessed by selecting **This Screen** from the **Help** menu.

From the **Help** menu, you can also select a **Quick Start Guide**, which will give you basic instructions on the functionality of the system. Review this before working in the system.

For a more in-depth introduction to the EHR system, select **EHR Walkthrough** from the **Help** menu. This document covers the various user roles within the EHR, their abilities and limitations, and steps to accomplish many of the key activities.

Hands-On Quick Start Guide

This guide is designed to help you begin using the system immediately. It is accessible from the **Help** menu by selecting **Quick Start Guide**.

The exercises in this guide assume you are logged on in the **Office (OFF)** role.

The Basics

Basic functions that you can perform within VariPoint EHR LP consist of:

- Search for patient records
- Sort or filter search results
- Create patient histories
- Update patient records

In addition to these functions, it is important to understand the concept of record ownership and the permissions of the different EHR user types.

Playing a Role

When you logged onto the VariPoint Electronic Health Record Learning Portal (EHR LP), you chose a class, then selected an assignment. An assignment has an EHR role within the ambulatory care setting, each with its own responsibilities, permissions, and limitations. This **Quick Start Guide** was written with the **Office (OFF)** user in mind.

As a reminder of which role you have assumed, the VariPoint EHR LP user interface has your **User** logon name and user **Role** in the upper righthand corner of the screen, next to **Sign Out**.

User Roles and Their Permissions

There are four roles within the VariPoint EHR LP:

- **Office (OFF)** receptionist, who creates appointments, adds and updates patients and checks in patients
- **Certified Nurse Assistant (CNA)**, who records a patient's vital signs and other medical history
- **Doctor (DOC)** (this includes registered nurse and nurse practitioner roles), who records patients' extensive medical history, creates notes and orders and signs them electronically
- **Practice Manager (PM)**, who verifies billable events for the clinic, such as appointments, immunizations, and orders.

More details about which role has access to which screens are available from the **Patient Appointments for [Day], [Date]** screen. Select **This Screen** from the **Help** menu.

Searching for Patient Records

Every screen with a grid listing of records has search capabilities on the right side. To search for a patient, do the following:

1. From the **Patient Information** menu, select **Patient Info**.
2. Scroll to the right side of the screen to display **Patient Search**.
3. In **Patient Code**, type "DWVPT."
4. Click **Search**.

All patients having a **Patient Code** containing the search criteria appear. These juried patient case histories come with VariPoint EHR LP.

To see all patients, click **Reset** under the **Search** area.

Sorting Data

Every screen with a grid listing of records has fields with sorting capabilities. These will help you organize your results.

1. Select "Patient Info" from the **Patient Information** menu.
    A grid display of all patients appears.

2. To sort your list of patients by **Date of Birth**, click the column header. All of the selected patients appear, with the oldest listed first. Note the red arrow pointing down.

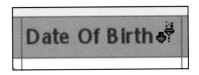

3. To show the youngest patient first, click **Date of Birth** again. Note the red arrow pointing up.

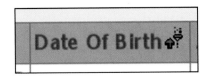

To remove the sort criteria, click **Reset** under the **Search** area.

Filtering Data

To narrow your search results further, use the filter feature. Different filter criteria are available depending upon the type of data.

To show only the patients for a specific family, do the following:

1. On the **Patient Information** grid view screen, click the bubble icon next to the **Last** name column heading.

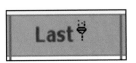

The **Filter** pop-up screen opens.

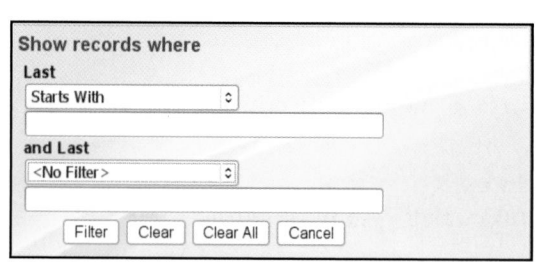

2. In the top **Last** field, select "Starts With."

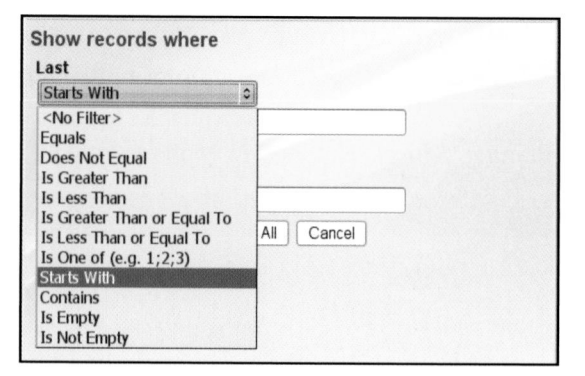

3. If there were other filter criteria, you would type that in the second filter box.

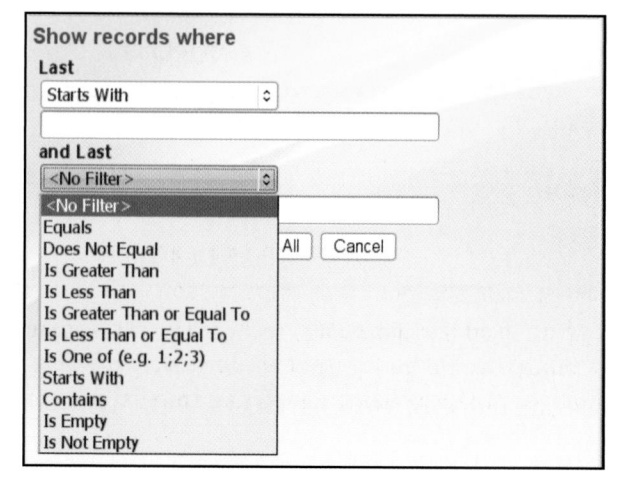

4. Type "Sakuramoto" in the empty field below "Starts With," and click **Filter**.
   All patients with the **Last** name "Sakuramoto" appear on the screen.
   If **Date of Birth** is the sort criteria, the results will be in birth order.

To remove one filter criteria, click the filter icon, and then click **Clear**.

To remove all filter criteria, click **Reset** under the **Search** area.

Updating Patient Records

Once a patient arrives for his appointment, an Office employee will need to update the patient's record with some minimal metric information.

To update your patient, do the following:

1. If your patient is not displayed, search for your patient.
   Click the tablet icon to the left of your patient to display his record.

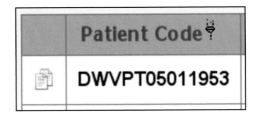

2. Click **Edit**.
3. Add the following information:
   - **Patient Code**,
   - **Date of Birth**,
   - **Gender**, and
   - **Ethnicity**.
4. Type either "whit" or "blac" in **Race contains (3 chars min)**, then select a **Race** from the filtered list.
5. Click Submit.
   Your patient's record with the updated information appears.

"3 chars min" Search

The **3 char min** field exists in many of the EHR patient records. By typing three or more characters in this field, you will narrow the selection results for a corresponding list.

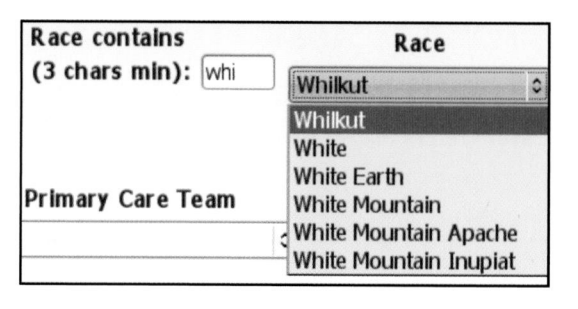

Owning Your Records

Record ownership is a key concept for the VariPoint EHR Learning Portal. The system allows you to update or edit the records you create but not the records created by others.

Your **User** name is on the screen. When you create a patient, the system saves the patient record with this name as the record owner.

To understand the concept of ownership and its effect on using the system, do the following:

1. Find your patient's record, and scroll down until you see **Patient Photos**.
2. Above **Patient Photos** are four fields:
    *   **Created By**, the name of the user who created this patient;
    *   **Created**, the date the user created the patient;
    *   **Updated By**, the name of the user who last changed this patient's information; and
    *   **Updated**, the date the user last changed this patient's information.
3. **Created By** should contain your user name.

Since you created the patient, you own him for the purposes of completing VariPoint EHR Learning Portal lessons. As a result, you can update this patient. The **Edit** button should be visible at the top of the screen.

You can also record other medical history information for this patient.

Now, find a patient that you do **not** own:

1. Click **View Grid**.
2. From the **Patient Information** menu, select "Appointments."
3. Click the tablet icon next to a patient other than yours.
4. Scroll down to see who is the owner, or creator, of the record. **Created By** should *not* contain your user name.
5. Scroll up to the top of the screen where the buttons are.
6. Note that there is a **View Grid** button but not an **Edit** button. This means you can see the record but not change it.

Common Error Messages

While working with the system, you may receive error messages. The most common ones are listed below:

- There is at least one issue with data submitted. See details below. This means there is a problem with your data. Look elsewhere in the record for a more specific message.
- The following field is required. This means a piece of required information is missing.

Need More Help?

Every screen has screen-sensitive help, accessed by selecting **This Screen** from the **Help** menu.

SECTION III

Guided Tour of the Basic EHR

This section guides you through the basic navigation functions of the VariPoint EHR Learning Portal (EHR LP). Steps are numbered sequentially, and screenshots illustrate key concepts.

This **Walkthrough** is accessible from the **Help** menu by selecting "EHR Walkthrough." The exercises assume you are enrolled in the Jones & Bartlett Learning DataWeb class "Training for EHR Learning Portal #DW-EHR-Training-100." If you are not, simply use the exercises with another class, choosing assignments that meet the user role criteria appropriate for the **Walkthrough** exercise. Section III, below, discusses the various EHR roles.

Document Conventions

To highlight key concepts VariPoint wants you to retain, the document uses several graphical cues.

✓ A white checkmark in a red circle indicates Key Learning Points you need to understand.

 An exclamation point indicates things to remember about the system.

About Electronic Health Records (EHR)

Electronic health record (EHR) systems are the electronic storage of patient medical information, including medical history, patient notes, and orders for procedures. They have several benefits. First, they provide decision support services for medical professionals and their patients. Second, they protect patients' privacy by segregating access to patient information based upon role and need to know. Third, they electronically interact with third-party service providers to exchange health and billing information. Finally, they provide healthcare providers and organizations the opportunity to determine and monitor health trends through data analytics. In summary, EHR systems offer an opportunity for increased efficiency, security, data analytics, and monitoring.

Process and Roles in EHR Systems

Within an ambulatory care setting, there is a distinct patient care and business workflow, from checking in the patient for an appointment, to the basic encounter with the doctor and other medical staff, to finally processing and receiving payment for patient encounters and services. The EHR encompasses those business process areas and segregates the activities into four roles:

1. Office Receptionist (OFF): Records a patient's personal and payer information and checks in a patient for an appointment.

2. Certified Nurse Assistant (CNA) or Medical Assistant: Records a patient's vital signs for an encounter (appointment) and other medical history.

3. Doctor/Registered Nurse/Nurse Practitioner (DOC): Records and codes a patient's medical procedure history and creates and signs notes and orders.

4. Practice Manager (PM): Reviews patient records for billing/payer purposes.

While some activities, or care records, are strictly for the medical history and patient health monitoring purposes, some events have financial repercussions.

VariPoint EHR Learning Portal

The VariPoint Electronic Health Record Learning Portal (EHR LP) enables you, a user, to use an EHR system in different roles within an ambulatory care setting. Now that you have received your logon name and password for the EHR LP, you can complete assignments using one of the four EHR roles.

The EHR LP will generate reports for your teacher and you with your activities, including the class and assignment, dates of activity, and actual values changed in the system.

Your teacher can review your reports online to assess your progress and determine if you have adequately completed the assignments.

Role-Based Activity within the EHR LP

The VariPoint EHR LP enables you to assume a role within the ambulatory care structure and work with patient data to that role's ability and permission level. The unique feature of the VariPoint system is its ability to provide two seemingly dichotomous functions: giving a consistent role-based user experience for all users completing a class assignment and at the same time giving you, the user, the ability to uniquely interact with your own patients' records.

To help you complete class-related assignments that fully utilize the EHR LP's characteristics, VariPoint has developed this **EHR LP Walkthrough**. The next sections go through key features of the EHR LP and explain the functions based upon EHR role.

Basic Functions of the EHR LP

Your teacher will devise assignments for your class that fully utilize the EHR LP's capabilities. These include adding patients, creating appointments, creating and updating medical histories, creating and signing patient notes and orders, and reviewing schedules for the day.

 One key feature of the EHR LP is its ability to segregate user activity while still providing the same experience. Fundamentally, each user *can* create a patient and edit her patient's information, but she *cannot* edit another user's patient's information. She can view that information, though.

CHAPTER 1

Office Receptionist (OFF) Role

The Office Receptionist role (OFF) has three main functions within an ambulatory setting and when using the EHR system:

1. Entering new patients and editing their contact and payer information
2. Creating, rescheduling, or cancelling patient appointments
3. Checking in patients

In Exercise 1 you created your first patient. Now you will create an appointment for that patient and check him in for his first encounter.

Exercise 1: Create a Patient Record

To complete this exercise, you will need the logon name and password you created to access VariPoint.

1.1 Logging On and Selecting an Assignment

1. Log on to the EHR LP.
2. The system displays the four EHR roles for the class. (Fig. 1)
3. Note that each role has its own distinct color coding throughout the exercises.
4. Click on the image for the OFF Role (Office Receptionist).

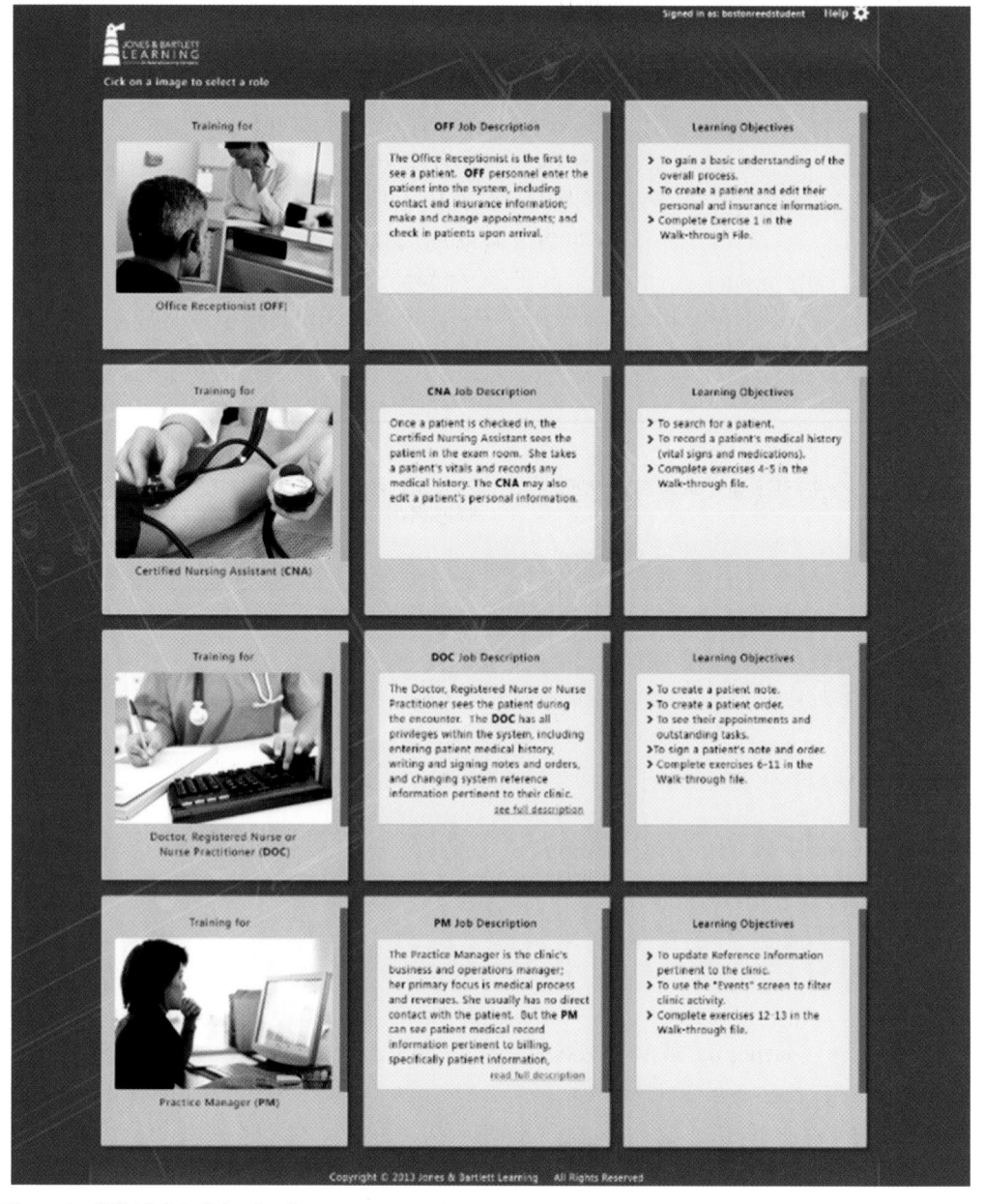

Figure 1   EHR LP Role Selection Screen
From this main screen, to choose a role-based assignment to complete, simply click on the image to select a role to gain access to VariPoint EHR in that role.

1.2 Understanding the Home Screen

1. The home screen is the base of operations for all EHR roles. Each role has a different menu and permissions options.

2. The OFF (Office Receptionist) role is the most limited, with only creation and edit privileges for patients and their appointments. They also check in patients.

3. Clicking the **Home** menu option returns you to the screen **Patient Appointments for [Day], [Date].** (Fig. 2)

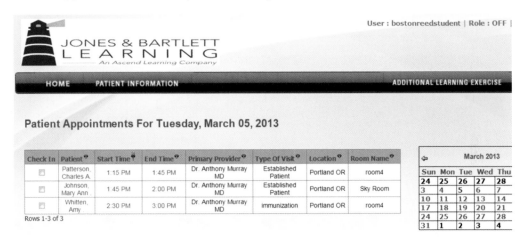

Figure 2 Patient Appointments for [Day], [Date] Screen
This screenshot illustrates the basic menu options for the Office Receptionist (OFF) role within the EHR. Clicking the **Home** menu option returns you to this screen.

1.3 Navigating the Patient Information Screen

1. From the **Patient Information** menu, select menu option **Patient Info**.

2. The system displays the **Patient Information** list, with **Patient Search** fields on the right side of the screen. (Fig. 3)

3. To sort the list data by a field, click the field name.

4. To filter the list data by a field, click the icon just to the right of the field name. Enter the filter criteria in the pop-up screen and click **Filter**.

5. To remove any filters of the data, click **Clear** below the **Patient Search** fields.

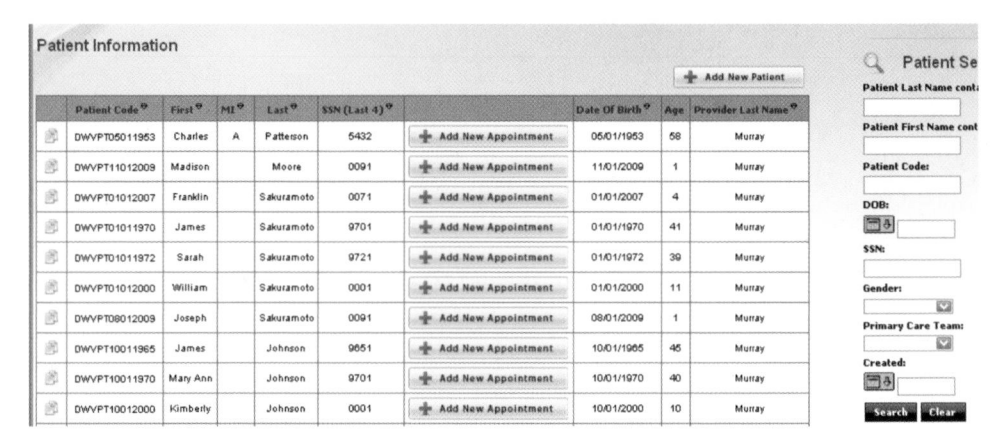

Figure 3   Patient Information List View
The screenshot shows the list of patients. From this screen you can add a new patient, add a new appointment, or search for patients. All screens with list view have search functionality.

1.4 Creating a New Patient

1. Click **Add New Patient** to add your own patient.

   The system displays an empty **Patient Information** form.

   ! The system requires several fields to create a new patient: **First (name), Last (name) and Primary Provider**. Most forms to add or edit information have required fields.

2. Complete the required fields for a new patient. Select yourself as the **Primary Provider**.

3. To uniquely identify your patient, give your patient a **Patient Code** (use the abbreviation of your college; for example, BCC plus all or part of your user id number).

4. Click **Save**.

5. Record your patient's information so you can find him later in the system.

   The system saves your record and displays the information. (Fig. 4)

> **!** Note the buttons on the screen:
>
> **Edit** enables you to update the record.
> **View List** returns you to the list view of **Patient Information**.
> **Add New Patient** opens a blank **Patient Information** screen where you can add
> a new patient.
> **Add New Appointment** opens a blank **Patient Appointment** screen where you
> can create an appointment for your patient.

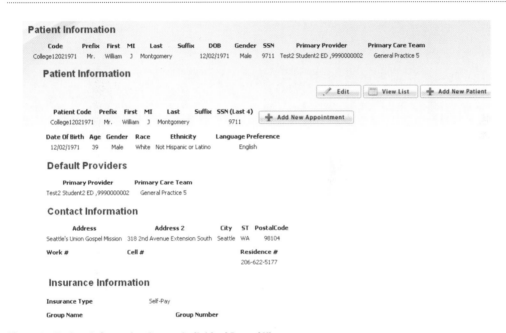

Figure 4 Patient Information Screen, Individual Record View
The individual record for a patient includes contact and demographic information, the clinic providers, and payer details.

1.5 Find Your Patient

1. On the **Patient Information** screen, click **View List**.

    The system returns to the list view.

2. Click **Clear** to display a full list of patients.

3.   Locate your patient by typing part of the patient's name or code in the **Patient Search** fields and clicking **Search**.

The system narrows the list to those records matching your criteria. (Fig. 5)

4.   Click the tablet icon next to your patient's record.

The system displays the individual record view for your patient.

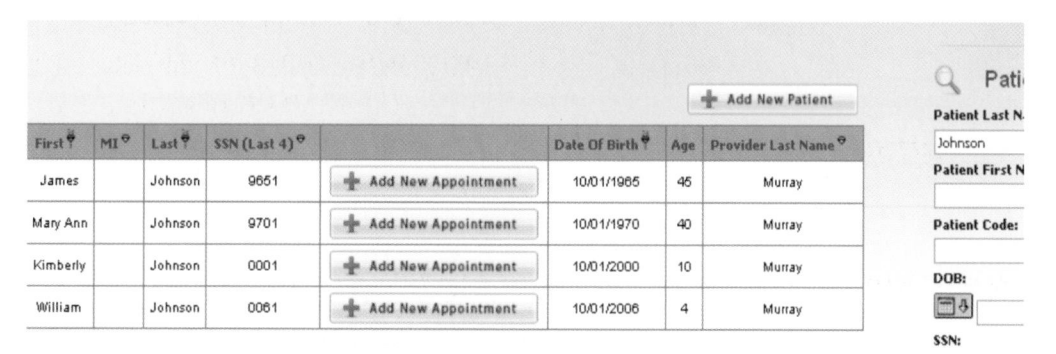

Figure 5   Patient Information Screen, List View Search Results

The search results for the **Patient Information** screen contain all patients matching the search criteria of **Patient Last Name contains** "Johnson." To start a new search, click **Clear** at the bottom of **Patient Search**.

1.6 Edit Your Patient

1.   On the **Patient Information** screen, click **Edit**.

The system displays the individual record in edit mode. (Fig. 6)

2.   Give your patient the following required information:

- A date of birth (**DOB**),
- **Gender**,
- **Race** using **Race contains (3 chars min)** to narrow the list results,
- **Ethnicity**,
- **Language Preference** and
- **Insurance Type**.

3.   **Save** the record.

The system calculates the patient's current age based upon **DOB**.

> **!** As you add more events, or care records, for your patient (appointments, medical history, notes, orders, etc.), the **Patient Events** grid on the right side of the screen will grow.

4. Return to the list view of **Patient Information**.

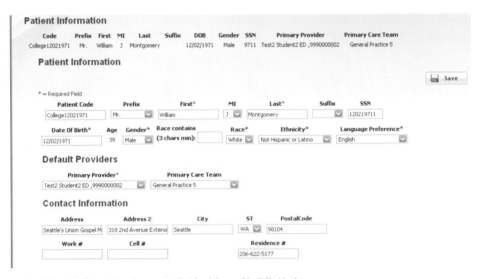

Figure 6 Patient Information Screen, Individual Record in Edit Mode
You can update a patient's contact and payer information on their individual record screen. Use **Race contains (3 chars min)** to narrow the list for **Race**.

1.7 Read Another Patient Created by Someone Else

1. From the list view, search for a patient whose last name begins with "Moore."
2. View his patient record.
3. Scroll down to the bottom of the record.

   Created By indicates another user created this record.
4. Scroll up to display the buttons.

> **!** There is no **Edit** to enable you to update this patient record. The system does *not* allow you to edit the patient's information because you *did not* create this patient record, e.g., you do not own the record. (Fig. 7)

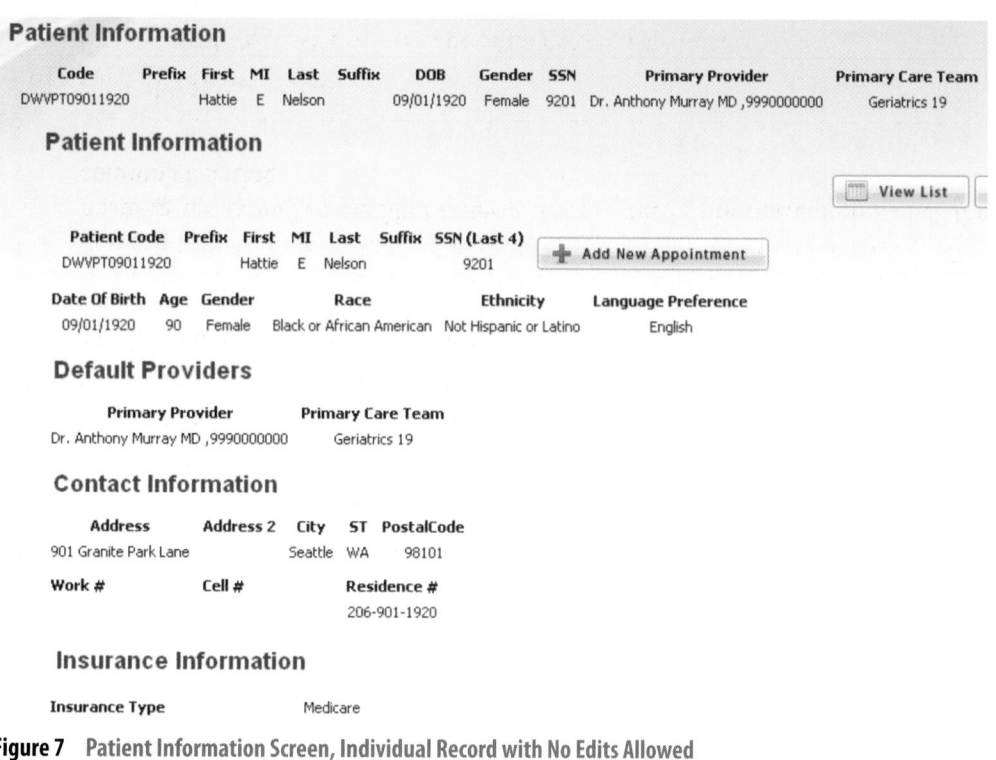

Figure 7 Patient Information Screen, Individual Record with No Edits Allowed
When you do not have editing privileges for a record, e.g., you did not create the record, **Edit** is not available.

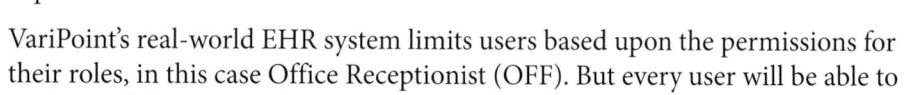

In the VariPoint EHR Learning Portal, *you can only edit the records you create*, regardless of the permission level for the EHR role you are playing. This enables the EHR LP to track each user's activity and maintain a unique yet integrated experience for each user.

VariPoint's real-world EHR system limits users based upon the permissions for their roles, in this case Office Receptionist (OFF). But every user will be able to perform all functions allowed by her role on all patients and their records.

1.8 Logging Off

1. Click **Sign Out** in the upper right hand corner of the screen.

    The system returns you to the logon screen.

You have just completed your first assignment!

Exercise 2: Creating an Appointment

After logging on to the VariPoint EHR System, select the assignment for the OFF role.

2.1 Add an Appointment for Your Patient

1. Select **Patient Info** from the **Patient Information** menu.
2. Search for your patient.
3. Confirm that this is the correct patient by viewing his record.
4. Select **Appointments** from the **Patient Information** menu.
5. Click **Add New Appointment**.

The system displays a blank **Patient Appointments** form.

> **!** An asterisk marks required pieces of information. For an appointment, several pieces of information are necessary: **Location, Start Date/Time, End Date/Time, Primary Provider, Primary Care Team** and **Type of Visit**.

6. Complete the required fields.
7. Select yourself as the **Primary Provider**.
8. Since your patient is new to the clinic, select "New Patient" from **Type of Visit**.
9. Click **Save**.

   The system displays the individual patient appointment record.
10. Select **Appointments** from the **Patient Information** menu.

    The list under the **Patient Appointments** heading lists the new appointment. (Fig. 8)

> You can filter the results of the list by clicking the filter icon next to the column heading and typing in the filter criteria. To sort the data by one column, click the column's heading.

11. Click the **Home** menu.
12. Click the calendar date of the appointment you just added.

    The grid lists the new appointment.

You have just created your first appointment. Bravo!

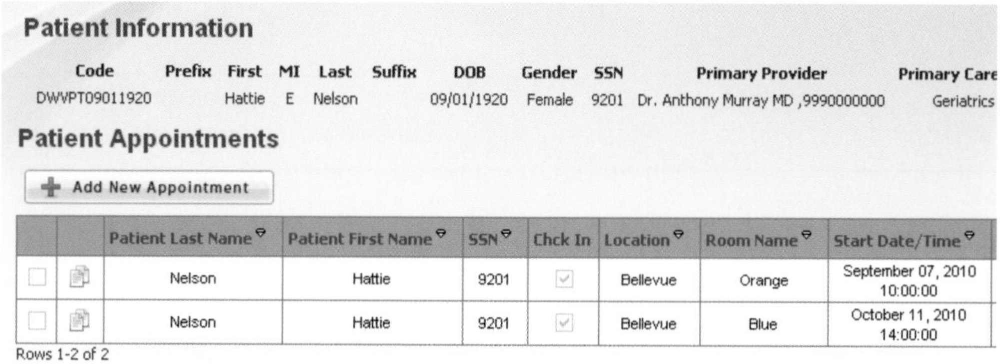

Patient Information

Code	Prefix	First	MI	Last	Suffix	DOB	Gender	SSN	Primary Provider	Primary Care
DWVPT09011920		Hattie	E	Nelson		09/01/1920	Female	9201	Dr. Anthony Murray MD ,9990000000	Geriatrics

Patient Appointments

➕ **Add New Appointment**

		Patient Last Name	Patient First Name	SSN	Chck In	Location	Room Name	Start Date/Time
☐	📄	Nelson	Hattie	9201	☑	Bellevue	Orange	September 07, 2010 10:00:00
☐	📄	Nelson	Hattie	9201	☑	Bellevue	Blue	October 11, 2010 14:00:00

Rows 1-2 of 2

Figure 8   **Patient Appointments Screen, List View**
The **Patient Appointments** list displays all appointments for a patient. Click **Start Date/Time** to sort the list by date.

Exercise 3: Check in a Patient

This exercise uses the assignment with the OFF role.

3.1 Check in Your Patient

1. Navigate to the **Patient Appointments for [Day], [Date]** screen.
2. Locate your patient's appointment by clicking the date for the appointment.
3. Select the checkbox to the left of the appointment.

   The other appointment checkboxes gray out, and a yellow **Confirm Check-in** button appears above the list. (Fig. 9)

4. Click **Confirm Check-in**.

   The appointment's checkbox has a check and is grayed out, indicating that the patient is checked in and the appointment record cannot be edited.

Now your patient can see the Certified Nurse Assistant (CNA) or Medical Assistant, who will record his vital signs and medical history.

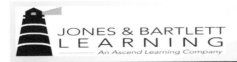

HOME   PATIENT INFORMATION   ADDITIONAL LEARNING EXER

Patient Appointments For Tuesday, March 05, 2013

Confirm Check-In

Check In	Patient	Start Time	End Time	Primary Provider	Type Of Visit	Location	Room Name
☑	Patterson, Charles A.	1:15 PM	1:45 PM	Dr. Anthony Murray MD	Established Patient	Portland OR	room4
☐	Johnson, Mary Ann	1:45 PM	2:00 PM	Dr. Anthony Murray MD	Established Patient	Portland OR	Sky Room
☐	Whitten, Amy	2:30 PM	3:00 PM	Dr. Anthony Murray MD	immunization	Portland OR	room4

Rows 1-3 of 3

			March 2
Sun	Mon	Tue	We
24	25	26	27
3	4	5	6
10	11	12	13
17	18	19	20
24	25	26	27
31	1	2	3

Figure 9   Patient Appointments for [Day], [Date] Screen, with Confirm Check-In
The yellow **Confirm Check-in** button only appears when you click the checkbox next to the appointment to check in.

You have now completed all exercises through the OFF Role!

NOTE TO USER: YOU MUST COMPLETE ALL PRIOR EXERCISES

CHAPTER 2

Certified Nurse Assistant (CNA) or Medical Assistant Role

The Certified Nurse Assistant (CNA) or Medical Assistant has one primary role within the EHR system: to record a patient's medical history and his or her vital signs during an encounter (office visit). In addition to these medical roles, the CNA can view patient information and appointment information.

The medical history components are limited in scope for the CNA role:

1. **Vital Signs**: They enter required vital signs during a patient's visit.

2. **Allergies**: They record any allergies to drug chemicals or other compounds (dust mites, fish, animals, pollen, etc.).

3. **Immunizations**: They record the standard immunization and date, selecting the manufacturer from an authorized list provided by the Centers for Disease Control and Prevention (CDC).

4. **Medication**: They record medications the patient takes, selecting from an authorized list of trade names provided by the U.S. Food and Drug Administration (FDA). These medications can be prescription or over the counter (OTC).

Exercise 4: Recording Patient Vital Signs

After logging on to the EHR LP system, select the CNA role.

4.1 Record Your Patient's Vital Signs

1. Search for your patient and display their individual record.

2. From the **Patient Information** menu, select **Vital Signs**.

The system displays the **Patient Vital Signs** screen with an empty list.

3. Click **Add New Record**.

4. Record the required vital signs.

   - A patient's blood pressure is divided into two fields, **BP Systolic, mmHg** and **BP Diastolic, mmHg**. Thus, a patient with a BP of 120/70 would have a **BP Systolic** of 120 and a **BP Diastolic** of 70.

   - **Smoker?** defaults to false if you do not enter a value.

5. Click **Save**.

   The system displays the individual record. (Fig. 10)

6. Click **View List** to display the vital signs for your patient.

   Based upon the patient's **Height** and **Weight**, the system calculates the **BMI**, or Body Mass Index.

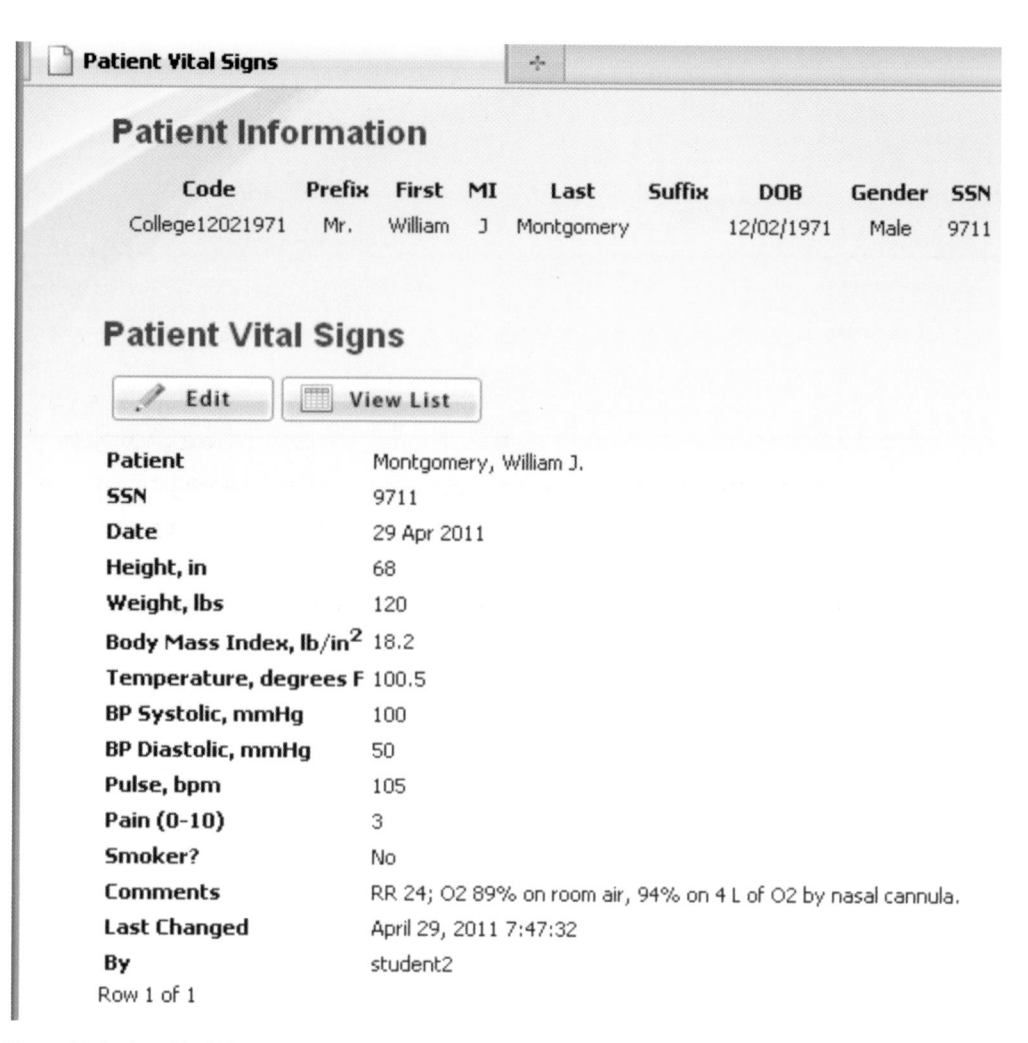

Figure 10 Patient Vital Signs Screen, Individual Record View
Patient Vital Signs screen displays the calculated **Body Mass Index, lb/in².**

Exercise 5: Recording Patient Medications

This exercise uses the class assignment for the CNA role.

5.1 Record Your Patient's Medications

1. If your patient is already displayed, from the **Patient Information** menu, select **Medication**.

    The system displays the **Patient Medications** screen with an empty list.

2. Click **Add New Record**.

3. In **Medication contains (3 chars min)**, type three consecutive characters of a medication's trade name, for example "Tyl" for "Tylenol." If there are drug chemical names containing the characters, the system will display those, also.

    The system populates **Medication (NDC)** with a limited list of drug trade names that contain "tyl" in the name. NDC is the acronym for National Drug Code.

 The system contains many **(3 chars min)** fields that limit the selection in list boxes. The more characters you type in the field, the more fine-tuned the results are in the list box. (Fig. 11)

4. In the **Medication** list, scroll down until you locate "Tylenol with Codeine." Select this value.

5. For **Status** select "Filled."

6. In the **Last Filled** date, select today's date using the calendar tool.

7. Click **Save**.

The system displays the individual record.

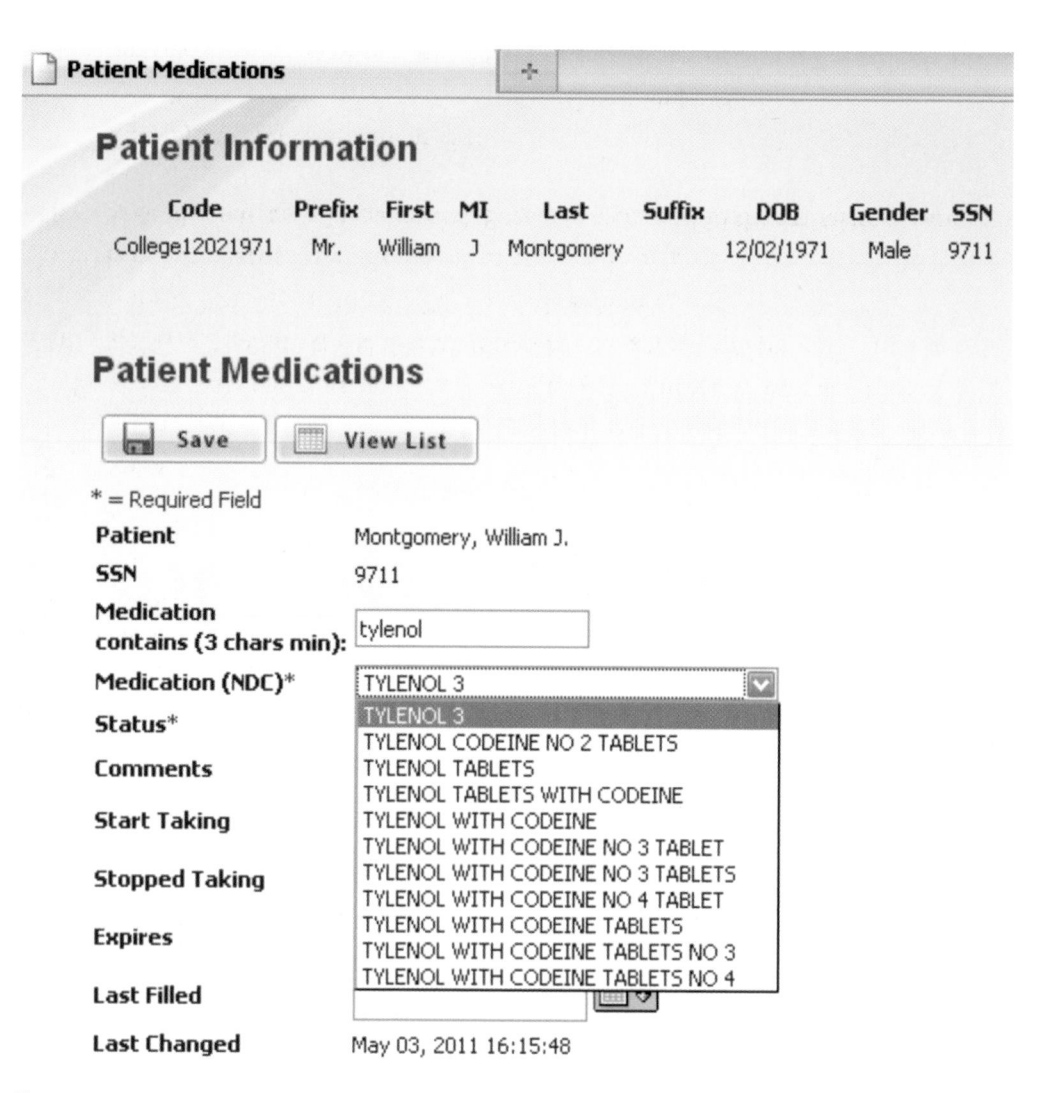

Figure 11 Patient Medications Screen in Add New Mode

The **Patient Medications Add New** and **Edit** screens have filter boxes for **Medication**. This screenshot shows the **Medication contains (3 chars min)** filter value of "Tylenol" and the list of "Tylenol" trade name **Medication (NDC)** in the list.

You have now completed all exercises through the CNA Role!

NOTE TO USER: YOU MUST COMPLETE ALL PREVIOUS EXERCISES BEFORE CONTINUING

CHAPTER 3

Doctor/Registered Nurse/ Nurse Practitioner (DOC) Role

The Doctor/Registered Nurse/Nurse Practitioner role (DOC) has the most extensive permissions in the system, other than the system administrator. In general they can perform all functions the OFF and PM roles can, in addition to several patient medical records functions unique to the role.

Specifically the DOC role has the *unique* ability to add and edit records in the following **Patient Information** areas:

1. Problems
2. Labs
3. Procedures
4. Notes
5. Orders

In addition, she can add new values to some **Reference Information** categories:

1. **Medication Status**: The filled status of a medication prescription.
2. **Note Titles**: The standard titles for **Patient Notes**.
3. **Problem Status**: The status of a patient's medical problem.
4. **Specialty of Cust's Department**: Specialty areas within the ambulatory care clinic.
5. **Visit Types**: Types of patient visits.
6. **Vital Signs**: Different types of vital signs for patient orders.
7. **Rooms**: The names or numbers of actual rooms in the clinic for appointment management purposes.

8.   **Primary Care Team**: Name and location of various teams within a clinic.

9.   **Primary Providers/Primary Care Team**: Primary Provider assigned to a Primary Care Team.

Finally, the DOC can view her schedule and unsigned notes and orders from the **Doctor Desktop** screen.

In the following exercises you will learn to create and sign **Patient Notes** and **Patient Orders**. You will also learn to read and use the **Doctor Desktop** screen to plan your work day as a Primary Provider.

Exercise 6: Creating a Patient Note

Patient notes include a medical diagnosis and the Primary Provider's assessment of the patient. To be effective, the note must be signed by the Primary Provider.

This exercise uses the class assignment for the DOC role. Log on to EHR LP, select the class, then select the assignment for the DOC role.

6.1 Record a Note for Your Patient

1.   Locate your patient and display the patient's individual record.

2.   From the **Patient Information** menu, select **Notes**.

     The system displays the **Patient Notes** screen with an empty list.

3.   Click **Add New Record**.

     The system displays an empty **Patient Notes** form with a **Note Date** having today's date and time.

4.   From the **Selected Title** list, click the standard notes title "General Note."

5.   For the **Subtitle**, type "Annual Physical."

6.   For **Urgency**, click "Routine."

7.   In **Diagnosis (or code) contains (3 chars min)**, type "V70."

8.   From **Diagnosis (ICD-9)**, click the code "V700."

> ! Code "V700" corresponds to the nomenclature for a general exam, "Routine general medical examination at a healthcare facility." You can also locate this diagnosis by typing part of the descriptive title. The more unique the text you type, the shorter the list. Try the words "examination" and "routine," and compare the results.

9. For the **Note**, type "Patient is in good general health."

10. Select yourself as the Primary Provider in the **Signed By** list.

11. For the time being, ignore **e-Signature**.

12. Click **Save**.

    The system displays the individual note record. (Fig. 12)

13. Write down the **Note Date** and **Entry Date** for later reference.

> **!** **Signed?** is "No" because you did not sign the note. The default value of **Note Date** is the date and time you started writing the note. The **Entry Date** is the date/time the record saved. Since you created a new record, the **Last Changed** date/time coincides with the **Entry Date**.

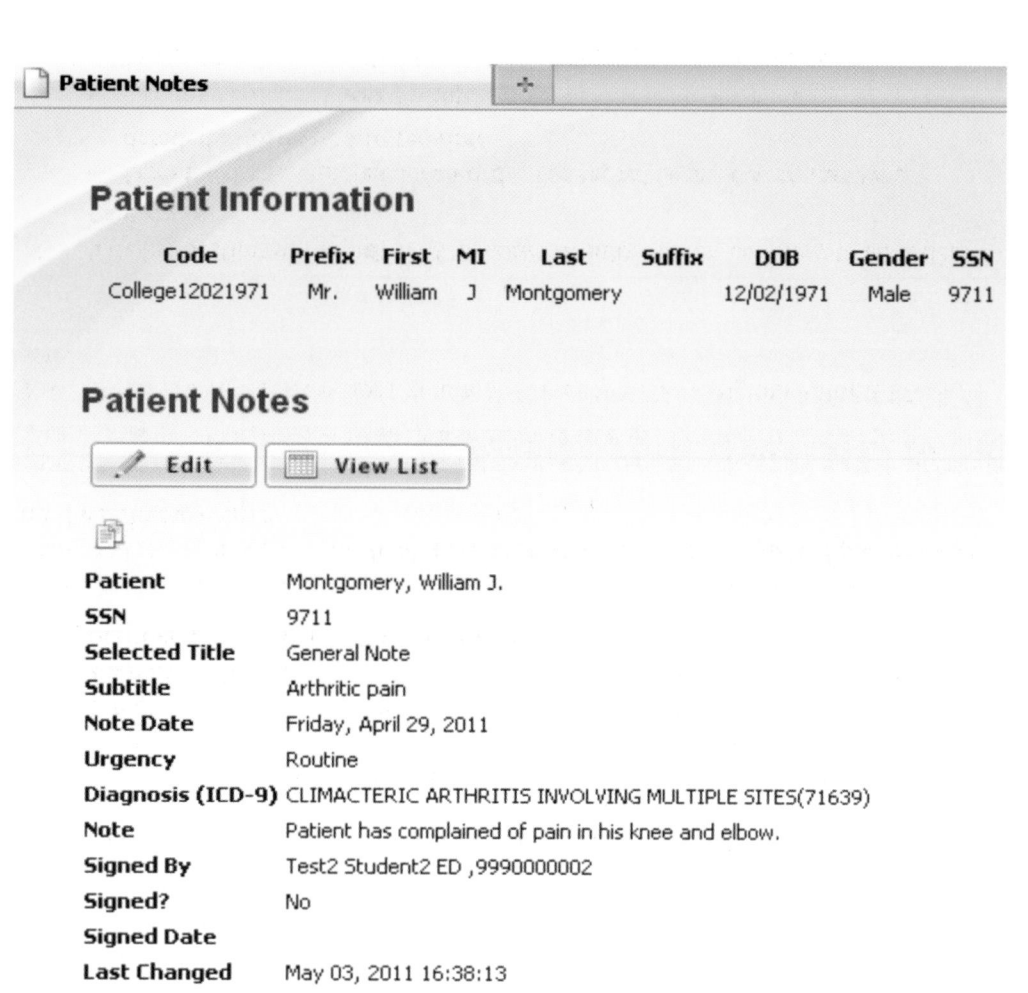

Figure 12 Patient Notes Screen, Individual Record
When you create **Patient Notes**, you must select a standardized **Diagnosis (ICD-9)** diagnosis nomenclature and code and type the free-text **Note** content. The system automatically records the **Entry Date** and **Last Changed** date as part of the record audit process.

In Exercise 11, you will sign your note.

Exercise 7: Starting the Patient Order Process

Patient orders include a medical diagnosis and instructions from the Primary Provider regarding the patient's care. An order can include a prescription for medication, referrals for procedures or consultations, lab tests or radiology exams, or specialized vital signs. To be effective, the order must be signed by the Primary Provider.

This exercise uses the class assignment for the DOC role.

7.1 Start the Order Creation Process for Your Patient

1. Locate your patient and display their individual record.
2. From the **Patient Information** menu, select **Orders**.

    The system displays the **Patient Orders** screen with an empty list.
3. Click **Add New Record**.

    The system displays a blank **Patient Orders** form.

 The orders process is designed to help the Primary Provider and Practice Manager filter information and track their patients' health more easily by categorizing the information. Based upon the **Order Type** you select in the **Patient Orders** screen, you can generate more than half a dozen different types of orders, each with their own criteria.

Let us explore what is common to all patient orders, the different types of patient orders, and their characteristics.

Exercise 8: Exploring Patient Orders

This exercise is a continuation of Exercise 7. It uses the class assignment for the DOC role.

8.1 Explore Patient Orders in General

1. The top section of **Patient Orders** contains information common to all orders (Fig. 13):
    *   **Order Type** designates which order the record is and determines what detailed information to require.
    *   **Urgency** indicates how promptly an order must be completed.
    *   **Order Date/Time** is the date and time the user began to fill the order.

- **Instructions** are the specific order directions. *Any details in the specific order sections must be entered in this area.*
- **Ordering Location** is the location at which the patient was seen and the Primary Provider is placing the order.
- **Historical Visit?** checked indicates this was recorded after the fact.
- **Primary Provider** is the designated signer of the order.
- **e-Signature** is the field the **Primary Provider** types her secret code for signing orders.

2. Scroll down to the bottom of the screen. The screen ends with **e-Signature**.

3. Select "V (Vitals)" from **Order Type.**

   The bottom of **Patient Orders** changes, displaying the specific fields for that type of patient order.

 Each **Order Type** has custom information displayed at the bottom of **Patient Orders**.

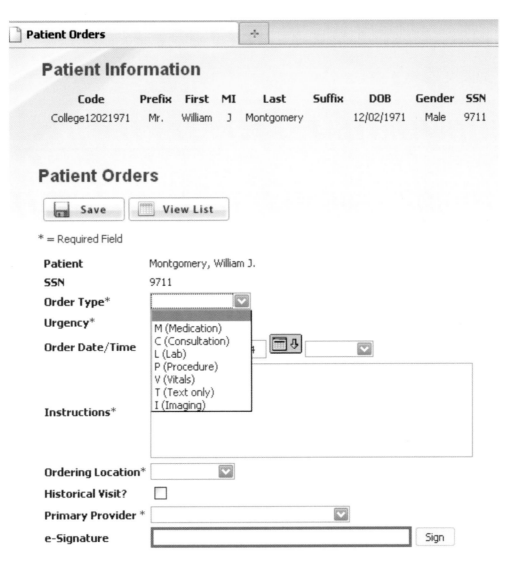

Figure 13 Patient Orders Screen, Add New Mode
Each order has common information, listed directly beneath **Patient Orders**. Every **Order Type** has additional information unique to its category. In this screenshot, the **Order Type** list displays all order selection options.

8.2 Explore Patient Orders for Medications

1. From the **Order Type** list, select "M (Medication)."

2. Scroll down to see the fields for medication orders.

3. A medication order is a prescription for a drug using the chemical name, such as "ACETAMINOPHEN," not the trade name "Tylenol."

4. Type "ACETA" in **Medication Chemical Name contains (3 chars min)**.

   Drug's Chemical Name (NDC) contains the drug "ACETAMINOPHEN" in the list.

5. A medication order also contains detailed prescription information, including the **Schedule** for taking the medication and pickup information. The select lists for **Dosage Form**, **Dosage**, and **Route** vary based upon the **Drug's Chemical Name (NDC)**.

8.3 Explore Patient Orders for Consultations

1. From the **Order Type** list, select "C (Consultation)."

2. Scroll down to see the fields for referrals to specialists.

   - **Disease Specialty** is the specialist's practice type to whom the patient is being referred.
   - **Attention** is the name of the specialist.
   - **Consult Location** is the physical location of the specialist, such as his or her clinic or practice name.
   - **Provisional Diagnosis (ICD-9)** is the ICD-9 diagnosis code that the patient's Primary Provider assigns to the patient—the reason for the patient consultation referral.

8.4 Explore Patient Orders for Lab Tests

1. From the **Order Type** list, select "L (Lab)."

2. The lab test fields available depend upon the **Collection Type** of the specimen.

3. Both **Collection Types** require the following fields:

   - Lab test (and number) LOINC
   - **Collection Date**
   - **Schedule**

4. If **Collection Type** is "Collect Locally," the Primary Provider types a **Specimen Description** and **Sample ID** for tracking. The **Specimen Date** defaults to today's date and time.

8.5 Explore Patient Orders for Procedures

1. From the **Order Type** list, select "P (Procedure)."

2. **Procedure (CPT)** uses CPT codes and nomenclature for referring patients to specialists for further treatment. **Procedure (or code) contains (3 chars min)** narrows the list.

3. **Provisional Diagnosis (ICD-9)**, **Consult Location**, and **Disease Specialty** serve the same purpose as they do for "(C) Consultation" orders.

8.6 Explore Patient Orders for Vital Signs

1. From the **Order Type** list, select "V (Vitals)."

2. A **Vital** is one of the vital signs listed under the **Reference Information** menu option **Vital Signs**.

3. The **Start** and **Stop** dates, combined with the **Schedule**, indicate the duration and frequency with which to conduct the vital sign test.

4. **Special Instructions** could include more specific directions, such as what equipment to use or what range of vital sign readings to record.

8.7 Explore Patient Orders for Images

1. From the **Order Type** list, select "I (Imaging)."

2. In the **Imaging Type** list, click "General Radiology."

3. The **Imaging Procedure (CPT)** contains the CPT imaging code groups primarily in the 7X000 series, including but not limited to the 75,000 and 78,000 series.

4. Type either a partial code ("781") or phrase ("xray") in **Imaging Procedure (or code) contains (3 chars min)** to limit the list in **Imaging Procedure**.

8.8 Explore Patient Orders for Free Text Instructions

1. From the **Order Type** list, select "T (Text Only)."

2. Free text orders have a limited number of fields—a large **Description**, a required **Start** date, and an optional **Stop** date.

> [!] **Description** in the free text order offers the most flexibility for Primary Providers to create orders. However, free text order types also require the least specificity, making it difficult to systematically categorize and track these orders.

Now that you have seen the various types of orders for a patient, you can complete an order for your patient.

Exercise 9: Completing a Patient Order

9.1 Write and Save an Order

1. From the **Order Type** list, click "I (Images)."
2. From the **Urgency** list, click "Next Available."
3. Select an **Ordering Location**.
4. Select *yourself* as the **Primary Provider**.
5. Select "General Radiology" as the **Imaging Type**.
6. In **Imaging Procedure (or code) contains (3 chars min)**, type "ultrasound."
7. Select "76977" from the **Imaging Procedure (CPT)** list.
8. Type the **Exam Reason**.
9. The **Request Date** defaults to today's date and time.
10. Type **Instructions** to the radiologist. Include the **Request Date**, **Imaging Type**, **Imaging Procedure (CPT)** code and name, and the **Exam Reason**. Add anything else you think pertinent, such as the patient's **Gender** and **DOB**, shown at the top of the screen.
11. Click **Save**.

If you completed all required fields (Fig. 14), the system displays the saved record. **Signed** will display "No," and **Signed Date** will not have a value.

Patient Orders

[Save]   [View List]

* = Required Field

Patient   Montgomery, William J.
SSN   9711
Order Type   I (Imaging)
Order No.   645
Urgency*   <Next Available> ▼
Order Date/Time   March 04, 2013 15:00:(🗓️⬇ ▼

Instructions*   Chest x-ray of patient
                       CPT 71111 X-RAY EXAM OF RIBS/CHEST
                       Suspected pneumonia

Ordering Location* <Bellevue> ▼
Historical Visit?   ☐
Primary Provider * Dr. Anthony Murray MD ,9990000000 ▼
e-Signature   [   ] [Sign]

Images

Imaging Type*   <General Radiology> ▼
Imaging Procedure (or code)
contains (3 chars min):
Imaging Procedure (CPT)* X-RAY EXAM OF RIBS/CHEST(71111) ▼

Figure 14 Patient Orders Screen, Add New Mode
The screenshot shows the completed fields for a patient **Order Type** "I (Imaging)" before you save the record. **Imaging Procedure (or code) contains (3 chars min)** contains "71111" to limit the list of choices in **Imaging Procedure (CPT)**. The **Instructions** contain the actual order to the radiologist, including the CPT code and possible diagnosis.

 In Exercise 11 you will sign your order.

Exercise 10: Using Doctor Desktop to Manage Your Patient Care Load

As a primary provider, you do many tasks, including seeing patients (patient encounter) and signing orders and notes.

This exercise uses the class assignment for the DOC role.

10.1 Read Doctor Desktop

1. Click the **Doctor Desktop** menu.

The system displays the **Doctor Desktop** screen. (Fig. 15)

 Doctor Desktop displays records for a user who is logged on to the system using the "DOC," or Doctor, role. Each category of information lists only records where the user is either the assigned Primary Provider for appointments or the assigned Primary Provider, or signer, for notes and orders.

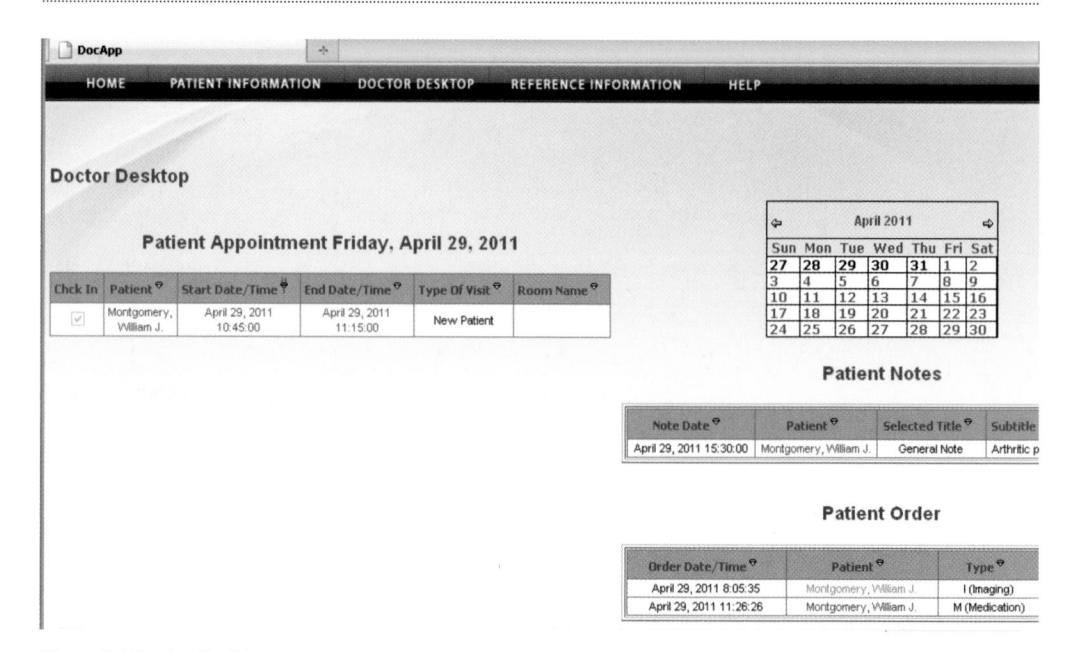

Figure 15 Doctor Desktop

When you log on using the "DOC" (or Doctor) role, **Doctor Desktop** provides you access to a list of patient appointments where you are the Primary Provider, as well as unsigned notes and unsigned orders where you are the designated signer.

2. There are three sections to the work area:

- **Patient Appointments for [Day], [Date]**, showing the Primary Provider's appointments for a specific date.
- **Patient Notes**, listing all unsigned notes where the user is the Primary Provider named in **Signed By**.
- **Patient Orders**, listing all unsigned orders where the user is the **Primary Provider**.

3. If there are no patients listed under **Patient Appointments**, select another date using the calendar to locate appointments.

4. Under **Patient Appointments**, click the name of a **Patient**.

The system displays that individual's **Patient Information** record.

5. Navigate back to **Doctor Desktop**.

6. Under **Patient Appointments**, click a date and time under **Start Date/Time** for an appointment.

The system displays the individual appointment record.

Exercise 11: Signing Notes and Orders

Patient Notes and **Patient Orders** are not permanent until the signing caregiver, or Primary Provider, electronically signs the record using her eSignature.

This exercise uses the class assignment for the DOC role.

11.1 Sign a Note

1. From **Doctor Desktop**, click your patient's name next to his **Patient Note**.

The system displays the unsigned note.

! An unsigned note has **Signed?** marked "No." **Signed** has no date.

---

2. Click **Edit**.

3. Type your **e-Signature**, and click **Sign**.

(Your e-Signature for purpose of this exercise will be the words **MySignature**. Simply type **MySignature** in the space provided once you have clicked on the **Edit**)

The system returns to the individual note record. **Signed?** now contains "Yes," and **Signed** has a date. (Fig. 16)

4.   Observe a few intricacies about the note's dates:

- **Note Date** is still the original date the note was first started (unless you deliberately changed it before signing the note).

- **Entry Date** (the date the note was first saved, not signed) has remained the same.

- **Signed** and **Last Changed** dates have the same date and time stamp.

5.   Scroll down to **Patient Note History** to read the signed note's record.

6.   Scroll up and click **Edit**.

7.   Type some additional text in **Note**. Type your **e-Signature,** and click **Sign**.

   Signed and **Last Changed** dates and times reflect the current time stamp. **Patient Note History** contains a second record.

8.   Return to **Doctor Desktop**.

   The patient note you signed is no longer listed in the **Patient Notes** list.

Every time you sign a note or order, the system creates a record in the history section of the screen, serving as a continuous audit trail and becoming part of the patient's care history.

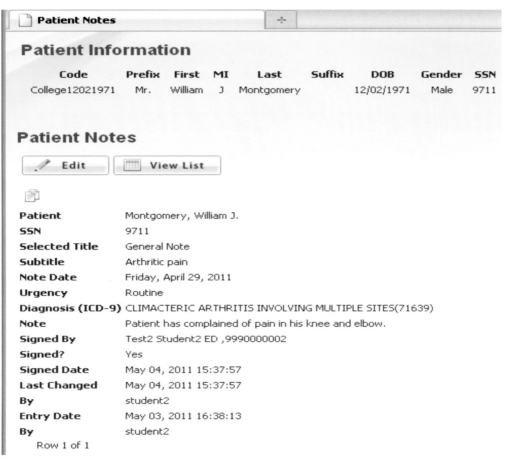

Figure 16 Patient Notes Screen, Signed Individual Record

The signed **Patient Notes** has "Yes" and a date and time stamp for **Signed?** and **Signed Date**, respectively.

The same process applies to a **Patient Order**.

11.2 Sign an Order

1.   From **Doctor Desktop**, click your patient's name next to his **Patient Order**.

     The system opens the unsigned order. **Signed?** is marked "No," and **Signed Date** has no date.

2.   Click **Edit**.

(Your e-Signature for purpose of this exercise will be the words **MySignature**. Simply type **MySignature** in the space provided once you have clicked on the **Edit**)

3. Type your **e-Signature**, and click **Sign**.

    The system returns to the individual order record. **Signed?** now contains "Yes," and **Signed Date** has a date and time stamp.

4. Observe a few intricacies about the order's dates:

    - **Order Date** is still the original date the order was first started (unless you deliberately changed it before signing the order).

    - **Created** (the date the order was first saved, not signed) has remained the same.

    - **Signed Date** and **Last Changed** have the same date and time stamp.

5. Scroll down to **Patient Order History** to read the signed order's record.

6. Scroll up, and click **Edit**.

7. Type some additional text in **Instructions**. Type your **e-Signature**, and click **Sign**. (Your e-Signature for purpose of this exercise will be the words **MySignature**. Simply type **MySignature** in the space provided once you have clicked on **Edit**.)

    Patient Order History contains a second record with an audit history of the second order signed. (Fig. 17) These audit records become part of the patient's case history.

8. Return to **Doctor Desktop**.

    The patient order you signed is no longer listed in the **Patient Orders** list.

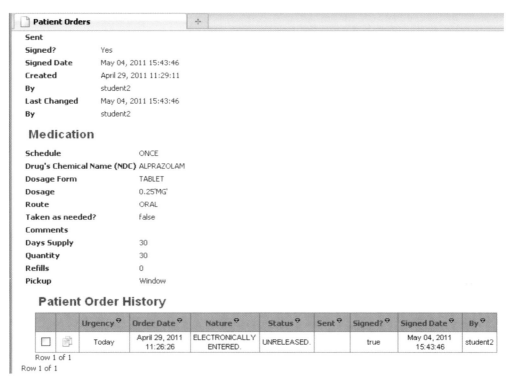

Figure 17 Patient Orders Screen, Individual Record with History List

Each time you log on to the system using the "DOC" (or Doctor) role, you can sign **Patient Orders** for which you are the listed **Primary Provider**. The system creates an audit record so Primary Providers have a **Patient Order History**, or case history, for each order.

You have completed all exercises through the DOC Role!

....

NOTE TO USER: YOU MUST COMPLETE ALL PRIOR EXERCISES BEFORE CONTINUING

CHAPTER 4

Practice Manager (PM) Role

Since the Practice Manager's role (PM) relates primarily to managing the ambulatory clinic and fulfilling billing, revenue cycle management (RCM), human resources (HR) planning, and third party contract management, his role is more limited in scope than the Doctor's role with respect to clinical care. But he does have access to some **Reference Information**.

From a practice and workflow management perspective, the PM will also be monitoring activity pertaining to RCM for the clinic—specifically patient appointments, immunizations, and orders for activities performed in the clinic. He can monitor patient activity using the **Patient Events** grid on the right side of the patient information screens and the **Patient Continuity of Care**.

Exercise 12: Updating Reference Information

As a Practice Manager, you will address management issues by updating the configuration of the clinic, both physical and with personnel. Your practice clinic has undergone a major remodel and added another treatment room. You also need to assign your new Primary Provider to two Primary Care Teams.

This exercise uses the class assignment for the PM role. Log on to EHR LP and select the PM role.

> As a user, you can add new records or edit your own records in **Reference Information**. You cannot edit or delete records created by other users.

12.1 Add a Treatment Room

1. From the **Reference Information** menu, select **Rooms**.
2. Click **Add New Record**.
3. Type a new **Room Name**.

4. Click **Save**.
5. Click **View List**.

Your new room appears in the list.

 The checkbox to the left of your record is dark, or not grayed out, because you created the record and, thus, are its owner.

12.2 Assign Your Primary Provider to a Primary Care Team

1. From the **Reference Information** menu, select **Primary Provider Care Team**.
2. Click **Add New Record**.
3. Select your name in **Primary Provider**.
4. Select a **Primary Care Team**.
5. Save the record and return to the list view.

   The list shows your primary provider associated with the **Primary Care Team** you had selected.

Exercise 13: View Patient Events

In this exercise, you will learn to see the activity for your patient.

This exercise uses the class assignment for the PM role.

13.1 Find Events for Your Patient

1. Under **Patient Information**, select **Patient Info**.
2. Locate your patient, and display his individual record.
3. On the right side of the screen, note the **Patient Events** list.
4. In the **Patient Events** list, click the **Description** for an "Appointment" **Event**.

   The system displays the individual appointment record for that patient.

 Since you are using the "PM" (Practice Manager) role, you see events that the PM role has permission to see—patient information, appointments, immunizations, and orders. If you logged on to the system using another role, such as "DOC," you would see events that the DOC role has permission to see.

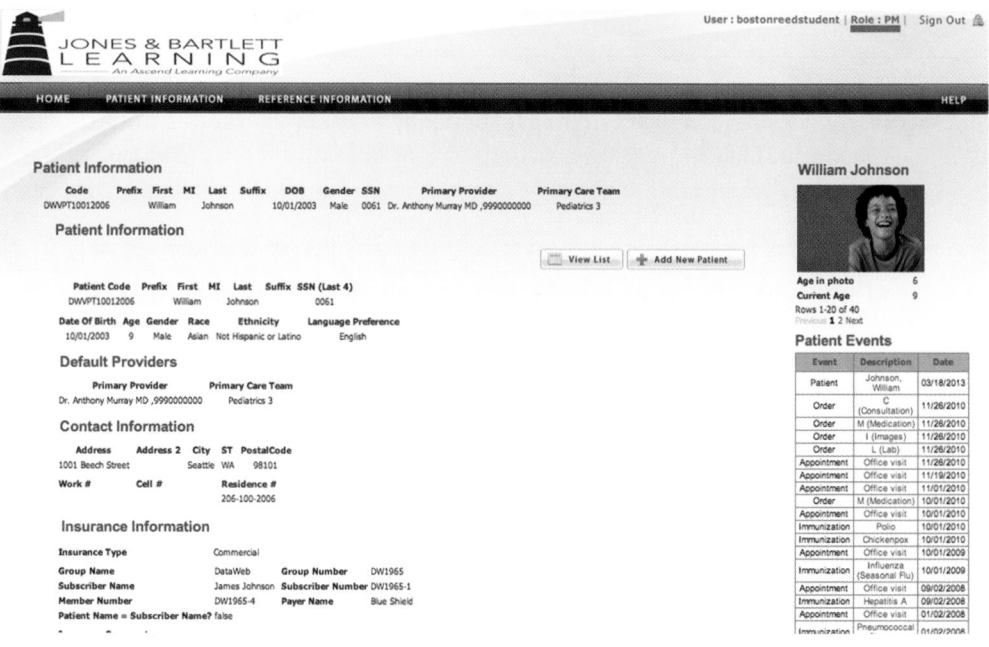

Figure 18 **Patient Information Screen with the Patient Events List**
When you create a patient care record in the EHR, the patient begins to accumulate activities or events. Any screen pertaining to a patient will display a list of his care records on the right side of the screen. The list will be in date order with the most recent activities listed first.

In addition to seeing a patient care history on the patient screens, you can find events matching criteria for your patient or search for the same activity for multiple patients using the **Patient Continuity of Care** screen. The system restricts access to care records based upon the EHR role you are using.

13.2 Find Similar Events Using Patient Continuity of Care

1. From the **Patient Information** menu select **Patient CCR**.

2. Use **Event Search** to find your patient.

! Since you are logged on as the Practice Manager, the system narrows the list of results to show only those care records to which the PM role has access. If you log on using the DOC role, you would see a more extensive list of continuity of care records because the DOC role has access to more medical information.

---

3. **Clear** the search criteria to display all records.

4. To check on billable events, such as appointments, select "Appointment" from **Type** under **Event Search**. Click **Search**.

The system displays all appointment records. (Fig. 19)

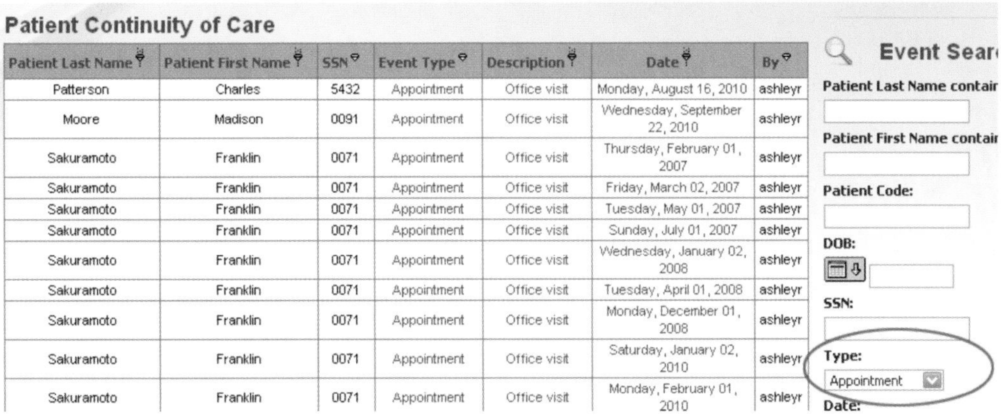

Patient Continuity of Care

Patient Last Name	Patient First Name	SSN	Event Type	Description	Date	By
Patterson	Charles	5432	Appointment	Office visit	Monday, August 16, 2010	ashleyr
Moore	Madison	0091	Appointment	Office visit	Wednesday, September 22, 2010	ashleyr
Sakuramoto	Franklin	0071	Appointment	Office visit	Thursday, February 01, 2007	ashleyr
Sakuramoto	Franklin	0071	Appointment	Office visit	Friday, March 02, 2007	ashleyr
Sakuramoto	Franklin	0071	Appointment	Office visit	Tuesday, May 01, 2007	ashleyr
Sakuramoto	Franklin	0071	Appointment	Office visit	Sunday, July 01, 2007	ashleyr
Sakuramoto	Franklin	0071	Appointment	Office visit	Wednesday, January 02, 2008	ashleyr
Sakuramoto	Franklin	0071	Appointment	Office visit	Tuesday, April 01, 2008	ashleyr
Sakuramoto	Franklin	0071	Appointment	Office visit	Monday, December 01, 2008	ashleyr
Sakuramoto	Franklin	0071	Appointment	Office visit	Saturday, January 02, 2010	ashleyr
Sakuramoto	Franklin	0071	Appointment	Office visit	Monday, February 01, 2010	ashleyr

Event Search

Patient Last Name contains

Patient First Name contains

Patient Code:

DOB:

SSN:

Type:
Appointment

Date:

Figure 19 Patient Continuity of Care Screen Filtered with the Appointment Type

Any patient care activity you record in the system appears in the **Patient Continuity of Care**. The **Type** to which you have access depends upon the EHR role you use when logging on. This example shows a narrowed list of patient events for the **Type** "Appointment," which is visible to the "PM" role.

Congratulations! You have finished the core Learning Exercises within the VariPoint EHR LP!

SECTION **IV**

Additional Learning Exercises

The Electronic Health Record (EHR) has been required for implementation through the HITECH Act of 2009. Included in the HITECH Act are meaningful use standards that specify what national and international standards apply to the various pieces of information gathered about patients.

In this chapter you will find a series of learning activities that are divided into two categories. You will find four lessons in the category of Standards and User Roles. Following this section, you will find another four lessons that focus on Patient Notes and Orders.

Any questions pertaining to patients within the VariPoint EHR Learning Portal use only the de-identified juried patients provided with the **Patient Code** having "DWVPT." Please search for this **Patient Code** phrase when answering patient-centric questions.

The lightbulb icon is a hint about how to approach finding the answer.

Category 1

Standards and User Roles in EHRs

Exercise No. 1: EHR Office Receptionist (OFF) Role

To complete this activity, log on to the VariPoint EHR Learning Portal and select the assignment for the role "OFF," the Office Receptionist role.

A. *Identify the standards used by the Office.*

What standards does the Office Staff use during the course of a work day?

 Be certain to check the **Help** menu under the Patient Information Screen.

B. *Identify the screen and data entry mode that uses the standard.*

During the Office process (add new patient, edit patient records, create appointments, and check in), at what point are the standards in Part A required?

C. *Understand the purpose of the standards and their inclusion in meaningful use.*

Who is the sponsor of the standards in Part A? How do they impact public health?

D. *Understand what encompasses the standards' families by using the de-identified patients.*

Name three patients who identified themselves as "Black or African American." Provide their names and patient codes.

 Be sure to check the Search Function on the Patient Information Screen.

E. Challenge Question: Thinking Outside the Box

Which standard is included as part of this EHR but is not required in the final standard for the HITECH Act of 2009? What was the reason for including the standard? Where did you find the answer?

 Consider the Insurance Industry in standards setting when discussing this question.

Exercise 2: EHR Certified Nurse Assistant (CNA) or Medical Assistant Role

To complete this activity, log onto the VariPoint EHR Learning Portal and select the assignment for the role "CNA," the Certified Nurse or Medical Assistant role.

A. Identify the standards used by the Certified Nurse Assistant or Medical Assistant.

1. What standards does the Certified Nurse Assistant or Medical Assistant use to create or update patient health information during the course of a work day?

2. What standards does the Certified Nurse Assistant or Medical Assistant see but not use to update records during the course of a work day?

B. Understand the purpose of the standards and their use in the patient encounter process.

1. Which patient has a temperature considerably outside the normal range? What does this imply?

 Be certain to check **the Patient Vital Signs** screen in the List View.

2. Who had a pharmacological reaction to a medicine for hypertension?

3. With which other vaccines is the diphtheria vaccine often combined?

 You might want to check the **CDC Standard Reference** website.

C. Understand what encompasses the standards' families by using the de-identified patients.

Has patient Robert Miller, DWVPT10011945, had any negative drug interactions? If so, which ones and what were the ingredients in conflict? What was the degree of the conflict?

 Check the Patient Medications screen report for DDI (Drug Drug Interactions). This is an example of how an Electronic Health Record can become a valuable decision support tool for the healthcare provider.

D. Challenge Question: Thinking Outside the Box

Which adult women in the de-identified patient set are obese? Provide their names and patient codes. How did you determine the answer? Provide the reference sources.

 Be certain to check the standards published by the National Heart, Lung, and Blood Institute (NHLBI).

Exercise 3: EHR Practice Manager (PM) Role

To complete this activity, log on to the VariPoint EHR Learning Portal and select the assignment for the role "PM," the Practice Manager role. The Practice Manager role is primarily concerned with clinic management and billable or revenue-generating events.

A. Identify the standards used by the Practice Manager.

What standards does the Practice Manager use or have access to for patient information and care during the course of a work day?

 Be certain to reference the HELP Screens that change, depending upon the screen. The answer is contained on three different screens.

What Reference Information that is clinic-based, not patient-care centric, uses national or international standards?

B. Understand the purpose of the standards and their use in the patient encounter process.

What is the age group that is immunized most often? What would be the purpose for tracking immunizations administered?

 Be certain to sort the **Patient Immunizations** based upon **Immunization**.

Assume you are a PM. If your clinic had pharmacy, laboratory, and radiology departments on site, what order types would you track and why? What standards do these orders use?

C. Challenge Question: Thinking Outside the Box

If a patient said he was from Europe and of Hispanic descent, what are the possible coding choices? What question(s) would you ask to clarify his origin?

Exercise 4: EHR Doctor (DOC) Role

To complete the activities, log on to the VariPoint EHR Learning Portal and select the assignment for the role "DOC," the Doctor role.

The Doctor role is primarily concerned with patient medical care, including notes and orders, and management of the medical nature of the clinic.

A. Identify the standards used by the Doctor.

What standards related to patient health does the Doctor use that no other role has access to? What are the screens? Why would these be reserved for the DOC role?

 Be certain to consider the special training required to use certain standards and classification information.

What **Reference Information** that is patient-care centric uses national or international standards and is only accessible by the DOC role?

B. Understand the purpose of the standards and their use in the patient encounter process

Which patients have transferred to your clinic with a previous health history and/or previous healthcare providers?

- Of these patients, who has the same diagnosis? What is the diagnosis?
  - What else do these patients have in common?
  - Why would a doctor care about what is common among patients with a similar or identical diagnosis?

What problems were diagnosed for patient Robert Miller, DWVPT10011945, on his first appointment with your clinic?

C. Challenge Question: Thinking Outside the Box

As of Franklin Sakuramoto's last appointment, were his recommended immunizations up to date? How did you determine the answer? Provide the reference sources.

 Be certain to check with the CDC website that is referenced in the **Help** Screen for **Patient Immunizations**.

Category 2

Patient Notes and Orders

These exercises introduce the user to the standards that the Doctor (DOC) and Practice Manager (PM) roles could encounter while creating and signing patient notes and orders. The standards herein are only a small sample of that found in the medical community and within meaningful use of the EHR system. The medical and business processes, however, are consistent throughout the patient encounter process, regardless of the number or scope of notes and orders addressed. The activities are designed to encourage the user to explore the system further.

This document is part of the class assignment for the "DOC" role.

Exercise 1: EHR Doctor (DOC) Role

To complete this activity, log on to the VariPoint EHR Learning Portal and select "DOC," the Doctor role.

The Doctor role is primarily concerned with patient medical care, including the creation of notes and orders for patients.

First, you will need to create your patient, give her an appointment, and record her vital signs.

A. *Set up your patient.*

Create a new patient.

Create a new patient with a **Patient Code**. The patient is a geriatric woman, African American and not Hispanic, who speaks English and uses Medicare. Give her an appointment for today, and check her in.

Record her vital signs: 5ft 6in, 140lbs, BP 150/85, pulse 98, temperature 98.7. She reports no pain and is not a smoker. Her oxygen saturation is 99% on room air.

 Start with **Patient Information**, and then move to **Patient Vital Signs**.

Provide the patient's name and patient code, along with the values you chose. What are the standards used during this process?

B.   Create a patient note and identify the standards.

Create a patient note using standards.

Create a patient note based upon her visit today with all required information. Include the patient's age, gender, race, and ethnicity. Include her vital signs. She complains of shortness of breath, palpitations and dizzy spells, which prevent her from gardening "every day." She had to move downstairs to sleep. She doesn't smoke and is retired. She has conjunctival pallor. This is her first doctor visit in several years, and an examination shows no other problems.

 When creating a record in Patient Notes, you may have to refer back to other patient information to create a complete note.

What standards-based information did you use to create the patient note? Include a copy of the text of the note.

C.   Enter your diagnoses.

Enter your diagnoses using the fields available.

Enter the primary diagnosis and secondary diagnosis using appropriate diagnosis codes and descriptions. The doctor's primary diagnosis is anemia. Another possible diagnosis includes gastrointestinal bleeding.

 You could obtain the code and full description for the secondary diagnosis by using a secondary online source and searching based upon the description. **Notes** can include a variety of information, including multiple diagnoses.

What is the standard used to code the diagnoses? Record the codes and descriptions for the diagnoses you selected. You may have to use an additional source to find the complete description or code.

What are the advantages and disadvantages to using a standard for a diagnosis?

D.   Choose a signer and save the note.

Choose a signer for the note and save the note.

Assign yourself as the note's signer, and save the note. Record the signer's name, the **Entry Date** and time and **Note Date** and time.

 Look for a dropdown selection for the signer of the patient note.

When creating or editing your note, what is next to **e-Signature**?

Why would it be important to select a doctor's name as opposed to typing in a doctor's name or initials in a free-text field?

E. Challenge Question: Thinking Outside the Box

Based upon the juried anonymous patient set, what would be some good choices for other **Selected Titles** for patient notes?

 Try using the de-identified patient data set from the **Patient Notes** screen in list view.

Where in the VariPoint EHR Learning Portal can a user add note titles? What EHR role must she be using?

Create a Patient Order

A. Create a patient order and identify the standards.

Create a patient order.

Create a patient order based upon the patient you created in Exercise 1. The order should correspond with her visit today and have all required information. She needs an urgent lab order for a complete blood count (CBC). Your clinic does not have a laboratory, so you will need to send her to a lab for the blood draw.

Assign yourself as the signer, and **Save** the order.

 Refer back to **Patient Notes** to find the diagnosis.

When adding or editing the order, what is next to **e-Signature**?

What standards-based information did you use to create the patient order? Save a copy of the order.

B. Create a second patient order and identify the standards.

Create a second patient order.

Create a second patient order based upon your patient's visit today with all required information. She needs to be evaluated for gastrointestinal bleeding. She needs to see a gastroenterologist specialist. The order should include the primary and secondary diagnoses. The evaluation is for a colonoscopy and an esophagogastroduodenoscopy (EGD). One location to which you consistently refer is the Madison Street clinic for PacMed. Assign yourself as the signer, and **Save** the order.

 Refer back to **Patient Notes** to find the diagnosis.

When adding or editing the order, what is next to **e-Signature**?

What standards-based information did you use to create the patient order? Save a copy of the order.

C. Challenge Question: Thinking Outside the Box

What other orders could the Primary Provider prescribe?

There are other possible conditions for the patient, such as new-onset angina, congestive heart failure, and atrial fibrillation. To help narrow the diagnosis and determine the condition, another recommended step is to conduct an electrocardiogram (ECG).

 Use the **Patient Orders** screen to examine the other **Order Types** listed.

What types of orders could the **Primary Provider** create to address these concerns? How do you indicate the test to complete on the order form?

Update Patient Orders

A. Understand the differences between the DOC and PM roles.

Locate the notes and orders for your geriatric patient.

Use the patient medical history screens to locate your patient's notes and orders.

 The answer to this question is not obvious.

Record the unique IDs for the **Patient Notes** and **Patient Orders** and their respective **Note Date** and **Order Date/Time**.

Use the **Patient Continuity of Care** screen to find your patient's notes and orders.

 The answer to this question is not obvious.

For the PM role regarding notes and orders, what patient information is accessible from this screen? How does this differ from the DOC role?

Record the order information for your patient visible on this screen.

B. *Change the patient order and save the record.*

Change the gastrointestinal bleeding patient order.

For your patient's order for examination for gastrointestinal bleeding, a better referral location for the patient is Evergreen Hospital.

Change the referral location, and **Save** the record. Record the value you selected and for what field.

C. *Challenge Question: Thinking Outside the Box*

What significant fields and/or buttons are missing from **Patient Orders** for the Practice Manager (PM) role?

Why do you think they are missing?

Signing Patient Notes and Orders

To complete the activities, log on to the VariPoint EHR Learning Portal and select "DOC," the Doctor role.

In the previous activities, you learned that the Doctor role can create notes and orders, and the Practice Manager role can update orders. The responsibility of signing notes and orders, or authorizing them, belongs solely to the Doctor role because he is primarily concerned with patient medical care.

A. *Manage your work day using doctor desktop.*

Find your unsigned patient notes and orders.

Go to **Doctor Desktop** to see your unsigned notes and orders for your geriatric patient.

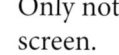 Only notes and orders that do not have an electronic signature appear on this screen.

Record the **Note Date** and time and **Order Date/Time** and the associated **Patient** for the notes and orders visible.

B. Sign your patient's note.

Using **Doctor Desktop**, select the note you created for the previous assignment and sign it.

 Use your e-Signature (remember to use MySignature as your e-Signature), not your logon id and logon password, to sign the note.

Record the **Note Date** and time, **Entry Date** and time, **Last Changed** and **Signed** date and time stamp information and **Signed By**.

Navigate back to **Doctor Desktop**. Is the note still listed? Why or why not?

C. Sign your patient's orders.

Using **Doctor Desktop**, select one order you created for the previous assignment and sign it.

Record the **Order Date/Time**, **Created** date and time, **Last Changed** and **Signed Date** time stamp information, and **Primary Provider**.

Navigate back to **Doctor Desktop**. Is another order listed for your geriatric patient? If so, sign it.

Record the **Order Date/Time**, **Created** date and time, **Last Changed** and **Signed Date** time stamp information, and **Primary Provider**.

D. Challenge Question: Thinking Outside the Box

What is the public law that addresses electronic signatures for patient privacy and electronic patient health records?

 Refer back to the introduction for some key topics to research.

What is the reason for requiring an electronic signature?

What distinguishes an electronic signature from a log on name or password?

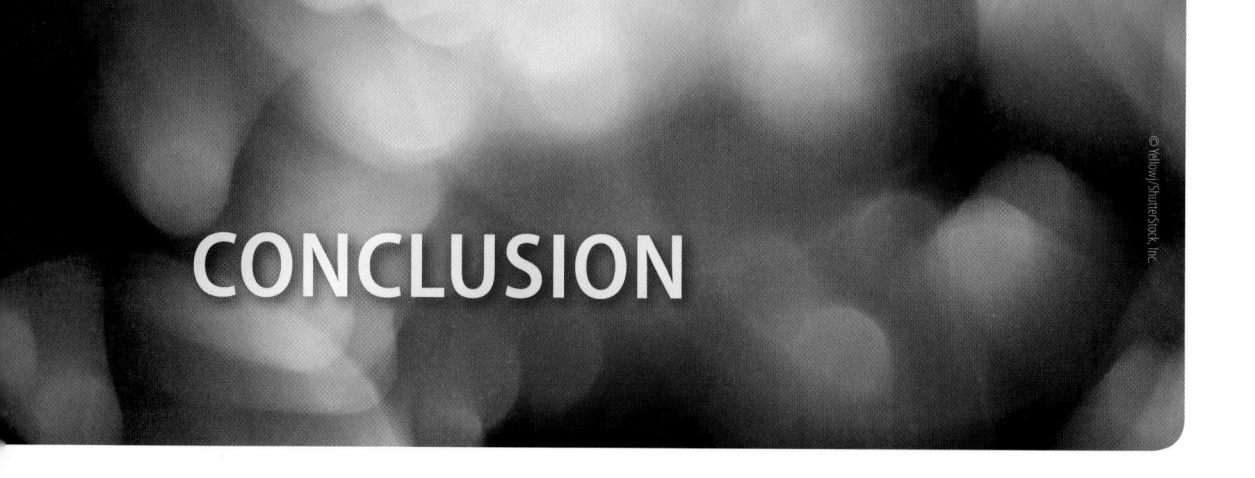

CONExCLUSION

The VariPoint EHR Learning Portal enables teachers to provide a standardized class-room assignment and assessment experience for the user. In turn, the user will be able to edit her own records, providing a detailed work history for the teacher.

By utilizing the four roles within the system—Office Receptionist (OFF), Certified Nurse Assistant (CNA) or Medical Assistant, Doctor/Registered Nurse/Nurse Practitioner (DOC) and Practice Manager (PM)—the teacher can provide a complete experience for users using an EHR system. And users can experience a simulated ambulatory care environment and patient encounter process.

Congratulations! You have completed all exercises included in the Training for EHR Learning Portal #DW-EHR-Training.

BIBLIOGRAPHY

"NSF names Bellevue College, HIMSS to open door to fast-growing Health IT job marketplace." Bellevue College, Washington [Previously Bellevue Community College]. Bellevue College, 6 December 2010. Web. 10 March 2011. http://bellevuecollege.edu /news/releases/archives/2010/NSFHealthITgrant12-3-10.asp.

Brokel, Jane, PhD, RN. "Moving Forward with NANDA-I Nursing Diagnoses With Health Information Technology for Economic and Clinical Health (HITECH) Act Legislation: News Updates." *International Journal of Nursing Terminologies and Classifications*. 21.4 (Oct–Dec 2010): 182–85.

Center for Health Transformation (CHT) and David Merritt, editor. *Paper Kills 2.0 - How Health IT Can Help Save Your Life and Your Money*. Washington, DC: CHT Press Publication, 2010. Print.

Fitzpatrick, Joyce J. "The Translation of NANDA Taxonomy I into ICD Code. Find Articles at BNET. CBS Interactive Business Network. *Nursing Diagnosis*, April–June 1998. Web. 8 March 2011. http://findarticles.com/p/articles/mi_qa3836/is_199804 /ai_n8798865/. PMID: 998731.

"How many codes do ICD-9 and ICD-10 provide?" DIMDI - German Institute of Medical Documentation and Information. DIMDI, 11 November 2009. Web. 21 March 2011. http://www.dimdi.de/static/en/klassi/faq/ICD-10/faq_0004.html_319159480 .html.

Joe, R. S., A. W. Kushniruk, E. M. Borycki, B. Armstrong, T. Otto, and K. Ho. "Bringing electronic patient records into health professional education: software architecture and implementation." *Studies in Health Technology and Informatics*. 150 (2009): 888–92. Web. PMID: 19745440.

Keenan, Craig. R., H. H. Nguyen, and M. Srinivasan. "Electronic medical records and their impact on resident and medical student education." *Academic Psychiatry*. 30.6 (2006): 522–7. PMID: 17139024.

Klehr, Joan, RNC MPH; Jennifer Hafner, RN; Leah Mylrea Spelz, RNC; Sara Steen, RN; Kathy Weaver, RNC. "Implementation of Standardized Nomenclature in the Electronic Medical Record." *International Journal of Nursing Terminologies and Classifications*. 20.4 (Oct–Dec 2009): 169–80.

Lynn, John. "Obama Wants Full EHR by 2014." EMR and HIPAA. 14 January 2009. Web. 18 March 2011. http://www.emrandhipaa.com/emr-and-hipaa/2009/01/14 /obama-wants-full-ehr-by-2014/.

Meyer, Geralyn, PhD, RN. "Diagnosis Development Committee Report: October 2009." *International Journal of Nursing Terminologies and Classifications*. 21.1 (Jan–Mar 2010): 44–45.

"NANDA List." EFN Home/Future Nurses. Eugene Free Network, n.d. Web. 21 March 2011. http://www.efn.org/~nurses/nanda.html.

National Drug File (NDF) Support Group. "National Drug File Support Group: Guidelines for Interaction Entry." Pharmacy Benefits Management Services. Veterans Administration, 1 March 2001. Web. 23 March 2011. http://www.pbm.va.gov/natform /National%20Drug%20File%20Support%20Group.pdf.

National Institutes of Health. "HIPAA Privacy Rule and Its Impact on Research." "How Can Covered Entities Use and Disclose Protected Health Information for Research and Comply with the Privacy Rule?" National Institutes of Health. 2 February 2007. Web. 15 March 2011. http://privacyruleandresearch.nih.gov/pr_08.asp.

"PubMed Home." PubMed. U.S. National Library of Medicine, National Institutes of Health, n.d. Web. 11 March 2011. http://www.ncbi.nlm.nih.gov/pubmed/.

Stair, T. O., and J. M. Howell. "Effect on medical education of computerized physician order entry." *Academic Medicine*. 70 (1995): 543. PMID: 7786378.

Toy, Eugene, MD; Donald Briscoe, MD; Bal Reddy, MD; and Bruce Britton, MD. *Case Files: Family Medicine*. 2nd ed. San Francisco, CA: McGraw Hill Medical, 2010. Print.

Toy, Eugene, MD; Robert J. Yetman, MD; Rebecca G. Girardet, MD; Mark D. Hormann, MD; Sheela L. Lahoti, MD; Margaret C. McNeese, MD; and Mark Jason Sanders, MD. *Case Files: Pediatrics*. 3rd ed. San Francisco, CA: McGraw Hill Medical, 2010. Print.

Toy, Eugene, MD, and John T. Platlan, Jr., MD. *Case Files: Internal Medicine*. 3rd ed. San Francisco, CA: McGraw Hill Medical, 2009. Print.

Voelker, R. "Virtual Patients Help Medical Students Link Basic Science with Clinical Care." *JAMA*. 290.13 (2003): 1700–1701. PMID: 14519694.

von Krogh, Gunn, MNSc, RN. "Taxonomy Committee Report." International Journal of Nursing Terminologies and Classifications. 21.3 (Jul-Sep 2010): 139.

Yamamoto, Loren G., MD, MPH, MBA; Alson S. Anaba, MD; Jeffry K. Okamoto, MD; Mary Elaine Patrinos, MD; and Vince K. Yamashiroya, MD. "Case Based Pediatrics for Medical Students and Residents." University of Hawaii. University of Hawaii John A. Burns School of Medicine, Department of Pediatrics, 2004. Web. 10 March 2011. <http://www.hawaii.edu/medicine/pediatrics/pedtext/pedtext.html >.

AACN Essentials of Baccalaureate Nursing Education (2008) – see ESSENTIAL IV – Information Management and Applications of Patient Care Technology

AACN Essentials of Masters Nursing Education (2011) – Draft from February which was just approved by the AACN Membership this week – See ESSENTIAL V – Informatics and Healthcare Technology IOM/RWJF Report on the FUTURE OF NURSING (2011)